CONQUERING CANCER

Dedicated to
Norman H. Olver (18/3/21 to 1/3/96)
who taught me the value of explaining things clearly

CONQUERING CANCER

Your guide to treatment
and research

Ian Olver

ALLEN & UNWIN

First published in 1998
Allen & Unwin
9 Atchison Street, St Leonards NSW 2065 Australia
Phone: (61 2) 9901 4088
Fax: (61 2) 9906 2218
E-mail: frontdesk@allen-unwin.com.au
Web: http://www.allen-unwin.com.au

National Library of Australia
Cataloguing-in-Publication entry:

Olver, Ian N. (Ian Norman), 1953– .
Conquering cancer: your guide to treatment and research.

Bibliography.
Includes index.
ISBN 1 86448 618 X.

1. Cancer—Popular works. 2. Cancer—Treatment—
Popular works. I. Title.

616.994

Set in 11/13 pt Bembo by DOCUPRO, Sydney
Printed by South Wind Productions, Singapore

10 9 8 7 6 5 4 3 2 1

Contents

Figures	vi
Tables	vi
Preface	vii

1	What is cancer?	1
2	What causes cancer?	23
3	How do you diagnose cancer?	51
4	Getting it early	74
5	How do you treat cancer?	89
6	The spectrum of cancers	137
7	Notable cancers	154
8	Prevention is better than cure	184
9	Treating the symptoms	195

Glossary	203
Reading list	213
Additional references	214
Useful Websites for information on cancer	216
Index	217

Figures

Figure 1.1 Shield on the Baltimore Cancer Research
            Center   2
Figure 1.2 The cell, chromosome, DNA and transcription   5
Figure 1.3 The cell cycle and cell division   8
Figure 2.1 Patterns of inheritance   26
Figure 3.1 Chest x-ray   63
Figure 3.2 Mammogram   64
Figure 3.3 CT scan   65
Figure 3.4 MRI scan   68
Figure 3.5 Ultrasound   69
Figure 3.6 Whole body bone scan   70

Tables

Table 5.1 Common chemotherapy drugs   107
Table 5.2 Side effects of chemotherapy   117
Table 5.3 Efficacy of chemotherapy   125

Preface

It was Francis Bacon who wrote, 'Knowledge itself is power'. The purpose of this book is to share knowledge about cancer with patients and their friends and relatives and so empower them to make informed decisions about their lives.

One of the great difficulties that patients have after the diagnosis of cancer is to be plunged into a whole new world of experiences with its own language and routines. A lot of information is thrust upon them in a short time so that treatment can begin promptly. I want people to use this book to gain a background understanding and to reinforce the new things they learn. By addressing the basic questions ranging from what cancer is to how it is treated I want to provide the tools to enable patients to ask their own questions.

I claim no special insight or wisdom, but I learned from the many people I have had the privilege to treat what they most often wanted to know and have tailored the information accordingly. As I wrote, I constantly found myself discussing topics and telling the stories of cancer and its treatment just as I would do when chatting with patients and their relatives. This book can be read to gain general information or specific topics can be found in the index and explored.

Cancer research is an exciting and rapidly expanding field which justifiably provides great hope to those people who are living with cancer. I have indicated the directions that research is taking and have tried to navigate complex concepts to share the wonder of the discoveries that have been made. Two experiences guided me in how I should go about this. First, my father was a lecturer in chemistry who successfully taught the subtleties of chemistry to medical students and expected clear explanations of medicine in return. This was often a challenge. Second, was the rebuke that I received from one of my patients when I was introduced on a radio talkback show as a cancer specialist rather than a medical oncologist, because the latter term was unfamiliar. She simply observed that the term would remain unfamiliar unless it was used, and I had missed the opportunity to do that. I hope that I have squared the ledger.

Mainstream medicine insists on basing treatment recommendations to patients on evidence collected in large clinical trials so that both the risks and benefits of the treatment are known. I regard this as a very responsible approach and one that those of us who are entrusted with the care of patients should adopt. I have tried to demonstrate the strength of evidence that is available on a range of topics so that people can evaluate any opinions they are given. Cancer is a highly emotive disease and there is a large amount of information of varying quality available. I trust that the knowledge gained from learning the evidence-based approach provides the confidence to sort the wheat from the chaff.

I am most grateful to my patients, colleagues and family who have provided me with the background and environment suitable for writing this book. I especially acknowledge the help of Jenny Olver, Graham Suthers and Jane Blake-Mortimer who reviewed sections of the text, Merrill Egorin and Vivian Hall who helped me with appropriate illustrations and my secretary Angela Casarin who, as usual, shared the responsibility of meeting the deadlines. I am indebted to Ian Bowring, the publisher who provided me with the challenge of this project. I have acknowledged patients, clinicians, family and allied supports, surely the same combination as is required to 'conquer cancer'.

Ian Olver

1

What is cancer?

Can'cer, n. The crab in the Zodiac; malignant tumour spreading indefinitely & tending to recur when removed.

—The Pocket Oxford Dictionary

When I was an oncology fellow at the University of Maryland Cancer Center, I often found myself drawn to the shield mounted on the lectern in the lecture room. This was no reflection on the lecturers, who were often leading cancer clinicians and researchers, but more a fascination with the symbol on the shield. It showed the claw of a large crab about to encircle a man's waist while he defended himself with a small knife (see Figure 1.1).

My problem was that it seemed the crab would win. This was certainly not the message about cancer treatments that it was meant to convey. What is the correct situation? To answer this we need to explore the frontiers of research into the causes and treatment of cancer where we will discover that significant advances have been made.

The term 'cancer' comes from the Latin word for crab because the swollen blood vessels around a tumour resembled the limbs of a crab. It is not bad symbolism—often, on x-rays,

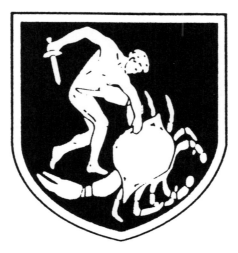

Figure 1.1 The shield from the emblem of the Baltimore Cancer Research Center of the University of Maryland

a cancer appears as a lump with legs invading the surrounding tissues. There are, however, a number of different terms used to describe this illness. We commonly talk of cancers, carcinomas, tumours, neoplasms or malignancies to refer to the same disease. If we define these terms we will be in a better position to answer the question—what is cancer?

TERMS FOR CANCER

First, the word tumour simply means a local swelling or lump. A tumour can be harmless or, as it is termed, benign. It doesn't have to cause harm by invading the tissue surrounding it or be capable of spreading to distant sites (the ability that distinguishes a malignant or cancerous lump from a benign one). As you can conclude from this, 'malignant' refers to those aggressive characteristics of infiltrating locally or spreading to distant sites which characterise a cancer from a benign lump. As for the term 'neoplasm', it simply means a growth of new tissue, which literally describes what a cancer is.

Carcinoma, from the Greek word for crab, *karkinos*, was the term for cancer used by the Greek physician Hippocrates. When used today it refers to the commonest type of cancer. Carcinomas are cancers that arise from cells lining the surfaces of the body or glands. Other cancers, such as sarcomas, develop from the connective tissues (i.e. muscles or bones). Also from the Greek is the prefix *onco-*, meaning a mass and signifying a tumour. Thus, oncology means the study of tumours. Oncology is also the term currently used for the practice of cancer medicine.

DEFINITION OF CANCER

It is important to realise that cancer is not one single disease. The term covers more than 100 diseases because there are many different tissues in the body, all of which can give rise to cancers. The causes of these cancers can differ as can the response to treatment. Any claims for a single cure for cancer, which treats all cancers as if they were one disease, need to be critically questioned. Cancers do, however, have some common characteristics. Their main common feature is that the cells that make up the cancer become abnormal and multiply out of control. To understand cells and what 'out of control' means we must briefly explore the normal structure and function of the body.

THE NORMAL CELL

All the tissues of the body are made up of cells. At the centre of each cell is the nucleus, which is like a memory chip in a computer. In the nucleus is stored all the information about the structure and function of the body that the cell could need. In fact, every cell contains the plans for the whole body, but only part of that information will be used by any particular cell, depending on its function. The nucleus of the cell is surrounded by the cytoplasm, a jelly containing all the processing plants of the cell. All this is enclosed in a membrane which forms the wall of the cell.

Unlike a computer, which stores information electronically, the nucleus of the cell stores information using a chemical called DNA (deoxyribonucleic acid). How DNA stores this information is fascinating. If you magnified a piece of DNA it would appear like two chains twisted around each other, with small cross-pieces (called nucleotide bases) regularly protruding from each chain and linking them together (see Figure 1.2). There are four different bases—adenine (A), thymine (T), cytosine (C) and guanine (G). A always pairs with T and C with G to form the cross-links. The varying order in which the bases occur along the chain forms a series of three-letter words.

For the words to be read, the chains have to unwind to reveal the string of bases; then a related chemical, RNA (ribonucleic acid), copies or transcribes the words by matching the bases on the DNA strand with complementary bases of its own. It then transports the message out of the nucleus to the cytoplasm's processing plants. Here the message is read. When translated, these messages are instructions for building different chemicals that the cell will need. For example, proteins are constructed from their component amino acids, or the building blocks of proteins. Each protein is made to have a special role in the future structure or function of the cell.

The DNA in the nucleus is not one continuous length but is divided into pieces of DNA, called chromosomes. We have 46 chromosomes. Twenty-three come from each parent. Twenty-two from each parent are almost identical, carrying information about the structure and function of the same part of the body. It may not be the same information—you might inherit the propensity for brown hair from one parent and blonde hair from the other. Which colour hair you will end up with depends on which characteristic predominates over the other. The 23rd pair of chromosomes, the X and Y chromosomes, determines our sex: if we inherit an X chromosome from each parent, we will be female; if we inherit an X from our mother and a Y from our father we will be male.

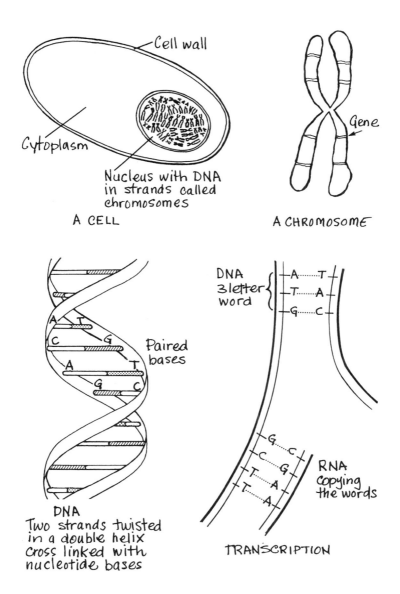

Figure 1.2 The cell, chromosome, DNA and transcription

5

Further, each chromosome is divided into blocks of information called genes. A gene carries enough information to make either a specific RNA or a protein that will determine a specific human characteristic such as eye colour. A human cell carries up to 100 000 genes, so that the information to make many products can be encoded for in genes.

The first cell of an embryo, which has inherited half its chromosomes from the male sperm and half from the female ovum, has all the information necessary to become a mature adult. It divides into two cells, then the two divide into four, the four into eight and so growth progresses rapidly. However, not only do the cells need to divide, they also need to start specialising, or differentiating, so that some become liver cells, some kidney cells and so on to form each organ of the body. At this time, although the cell still has the plan for the whole body, certain pieces of information that a particular cell won't need can be switched off. There also have to be commands that tell the cells when to stop dividing, or there would be an overgrowth of one tissue at the expense of another. When cells become highly specialised they lose their capacity to divide but, within each organ, there always remain more primitive cells, called stem cells, which retain their capacity to divide so that any damaged cells can be replaced.

Essentially, the processes of cell division and differentiation depend on some of the genes in a cell being switched on and some switched off. When switched on, a gene is said to be 'expressed'. This means that the chemical or protein that it codes for is allowed to be made. The whole process of regulating the genes relies on chemicals carrying messages about cell division and specialisation from one cell to the next. These chemicals, of course, were originally the products of other genes, so the regulatory process is a complex balancing act.

The cell cycle

At any one time, most cells in the body are resting. However, they can move from the resting phase and enter a cell cycle

6

which ends with the cell dividing into two daughter cells. There are several phases to this cycle—there is a time when RNA and proteins are being manufactured, and a time when DNA is copied so that each daughter cell will have a complete copy of the DNA with all the information it contains. After copying, one copy of each chromosome is pulled by a protein spindle to each end of the cell in a process called mitosis. The spindle is made of protein fibres that stretch from one end of a cell to the other. The chromosomes attach themselves near the centre of the spindle and are drawn towards each end of the cell as the spindle fibres contract. When complete there is a copy of all the chromosomes at each end of the cell and it can divide into two daughter cells (see Figure 1.3).

Controlling cell division

In a fully developed adult, the many cells in the various organs of the body that are no longer dividing, but in a resting state, can be stimulated to resume dividing by external chemical signals. This will happen if the body needs to produce more cells—for example, when there is need to repair a part of the body after an accident. These chemicals, which come from outside the cell and control the life cycle of the cell by telling it when to divide, are known as mitogens. Growth factors, produced by cells to act on their neighbouring cells, are one type of mitogen. Other mitogens include hormones, or chemical messengers, which can be produced in one organ of the body and circulate to distant parts of the body. This enables the growth of each cell to fit into the game plan of the whole body. Mitogens from outside the cell can activate a chain of events inside the cell. This is called signal transduction. The mitogen contacts receptors on the wall of the cell. This process is very like a key (the mitogen) fitting into its lock (the receptor). It triggers a series of signals which reach the nucleus of the cell with the message to start the process that will lead to the cell dividing.

The interaction at the nucleus with the DNA bases of a gene can alter whether that gene is expressed. New techniques

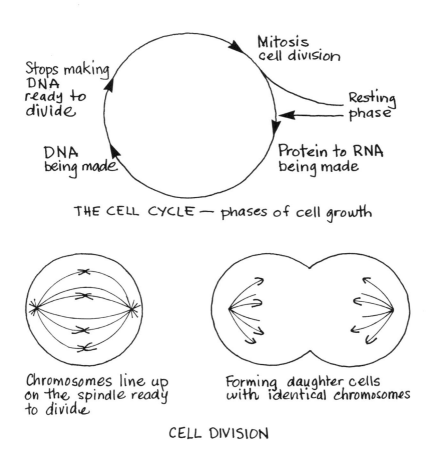

Stops making
DNA
ready to
divide

Mitosis
cell division

Resting
phase

DNA
being made

Protein to RNA
being made

THE CELL CYCLE — phases of cell growth

Chromosomes line up
on the spindle ready
to divide

Forming daughter cells
with identical chromosomes

CELL DIVISION

Figure 1.3 The cell cycle and cell division

have enabled the biology of these interactions to be studied at
the molecular level. Understanding what normally occurs in
regulating these processes can lead to discovering what goes
wrong in cancer and may, in future, allow us to correct these
faults.

Mutations

Cancer occurs because of changes to a cell's DNA. These changes, called mutations, alter the message coded in the DNA. This creates an abnormal plan for differentiation and proliferation for that cell but, worse, the abnormality is passed on to all the daughter cells at the time of cell division. The DNA can be changed from normal by chemicals or radiation. Viruses can disrupt the genetic message by inserting pieces of their DNA into the cell's DNA. Cells altered by these changes may not function. They may keep growing instead of differentiating or they may not be able to recognise the signals that tell them when to die.

It is worth highlighting, at this stage, that the development of a cancer, a process known as carcinogenesis, is a multi-step process. Usually multiple alterations in the DNA of genes of a cell occur over several years. The first event altering the DNA may initiate the process but further insults must occur to promote the process so that a cancer is produced. Cells can repair defects in the DNA but, if this doesn't occur, there will be a cumulative effect of DNA damage on the control of a cell's ability to grow, divide or differentiate.

Another way that DNA can become disrupted occurs at the time of division. Sometimes when a cell divides the chromosomes don't split properly. Pieces of one chromosome may break and join to another chromosome. This disrupts the normal message sequence encoded in the DNA, which we discussed earlier, and can lead to the overproduction of proteins such as growth factors, which in turn can cause the uncontrolled growth of cells.

There are several genes in the normal cell which, if altered, are most likely to result in cancer. They are called oncogenes.

Oncogenes

It may seem surprising that normal cells contain oncogenes since the word translates as 'cancer-causing genes'. Strictly, these normal genes are known as proto-oncogenes, indicating that they come from the body but have the potential to cause cancer. Why does the body have this type of gene? Obviously, they are not there to cause cancer. In the normal cell, the products of these genes are involved in the regulation of the cell's proliferation and only under abnormal conditions will these genes be turned on inappropriately. Because the normal function of oncogenes is to be part of the cell division process when needed, and because growth is not common in many organs after they mature, these genes must be closely regulated. If they are switched on inappropriately, malignant growth can result. Oncogenes that are inappropriately stimulated can eliminate the need for external factors to initiate the signal that tells the cell to divide. The cell then becomes independent of the outside factors, which are meant to be produced to cause the cell to divide only when the rest of the body needs it to.

There are several possible ways in which an oncogene can be inappropriately activated. The cell's own proto-oncogene can become altered or mutated so that the protein it produces is abnormal and behaves abnormally. The cell can become infected with a virus, which is just a small packet of genetic material, and this may contain an oncogene. Oncogenic viruses may contain DNA or RNA which can cause tumours to form when inserted into a cell. DNA from viruses can encode for proteins which interact with the chemicals in cells that regulate growth. The RNA viruses can result in oncogene sequences being added to the cell's genes or they can cause overexpression of the cell's oncogene protein so that too much is produced. In some tumours, oncogenes are found to have been duplicated or amplified, although how this happens is unclear. This results in uncontrolled growth—in other words, cancer.

Tumour suppressor genes

Tumour suppressor genes are also part of the normal cell's DNA, but with an opposite function to that of oncogenes. Their job is to suppress growth. As part of the normal functioning of the body, old cells will die and be replaced. These cells are programmed to die, a process called apoptosis, and tumour suppressor genes, through the products they instruct the cell to make, ensure that cells die when their time has come. They also take a part in regulating phases of the cell cycle and are involved in the signalling pathways that control cell division. In these functions there is a balance between proto-oncogenes and tumour suppressor genes.

We can see from this that loss, mutation or inactivation of a tumour suppressor gene could initiate the process that transforms a cell into a cancer cell, which does not die when it should. Understanding the fine control of this process is currently a significant area of basic cancer research. It may help us to increase our understanding of how our current anti-cancer treatments work and provide targets for more novel therapies.

THE GROWTH OF CANCERS

Even in cancers, the cells that are actively dividing at any one time are in the minority, usually less than 10 per cent. This growth fraction, however, is higher than in many normal tissues. The remaining cells are in a resting phase. The rate at which a cancer grows is not constant over its lifetime. Experiments have shown that in the early part of its growth the tumour grows quickly and the growth fraction is high. As the cancer becomes larger, its rate of growth slows and the percentage of cells that are in the cell cycle and dividing becomes less. The time a tumour takes to double in volume becomes greater as the tumour becomes larger. This is because more cells die as the tumour starts to outgrow its blood supply and some of its cells differentiate and lose their capacity to divide, just as specialised cells do in normal tissues.

Much of the growth of a tumour occurs before we can detect it clinically—that is, either by feeling a lump or seeing it on an x-ray. It is usually considered that a tumour needs to have reached the size of a cubic centimetre to be clinically detectable, at which stage it contains a billion (10^9) cells and weighs 1 gram! In the ideal case, it would take 30 doublings from the first cancer cell to reach this size. Ten more doublings and the tumour would reach 1 kilogram of tissue, which is usually considered lethal. These numbers tell us that, in dealing with clinically detectable tumours, we are operating at the tip of the iceberg. The tumour has already been growing for a considerable time before it is detected, thus shortening the time before it overwhelms the individual.

The doubling times of cancers cover a wide range. At one end of the scale is a fast-growing cancer known as Burkitt's lymphoma, where the doubling time has been recorded at less than three days. Conversely, some of the bowel cancers have doubling times of more than 600 days and would therefore appear to grow very slowly. Even within a group of similar types of bowel cancers there can be a large range of doubling times, making it difficult to predict accurately the aggressiveness of an individual's cancer. With this great span of tumour growth rates, we must be very careful in evaluating any new therapy to ensure that the treatment is altering the course of the disease and not just appearing to do well because the tumour has a favourable natural history with a long doubling time. We return to issues affecting the design of clinical trials when we discuss the range of treatments available (Chapter 5).

The doubling times also mean that most solid tumours have been growing for about two years by the time they are detected. This has important implications for determining the cause of a cancer, since events that occur just before the detection of a cancer are not going to be what caused it. For this reason, some patients' strongly held beliefs about the cause of their cancer can be discounted. It is common for people to try to relate the discovery of their cancer to a recognisable, often unpleasant event. An emotionally stressful incident is one example, but more often physical trauma is blamed.

'I was playing tennis and was hit in the breast by a tennis ball. My breast became sore and I found a lump.' 'I was playing football and was kicked in the groin. Soon afterwards I found a hard lump in my testicle.' These are common stories. In both these cases, the cancer would have been growing for months, if not years, before the injury occurred. The trauma served merely to draw attention to the body area involved and the cancer was then detected. Until then it may have been present without pain or other symptoms. The trauma had no part in causing the cancer.

WHERE IS THE IMMUNE SYSTEM WHEN YOU NEED IT?

The body has an immune defence system, consisting of two parts. One part uses circulating proteins called antibodies to identify foreign targets or antigens. The other part mobilises the type of white blood cells known as lymphocytes to attack invading cells or infective agents. Both these activities could be useful in fighting cancer, but one of the problems with cancer is that, unlike infection, it is derived from the body's own cells and may not be recognised as foreign. Some differences are apparent, related to the proteins or antigens on the cell surface, and these may allow the host body to mount a response. We see later how these antigens may be utilised as targets for therapy. Once the tumour is visible, however, it has probably overwhelmed the immune system and will need to be reduced in size by other means.

It is clear that an immune attack on cancer cells will need to be mounted specifically against those cells. Non-specific attempts to stimulate the immune system generally—often advocated as part of unorthodox treatments—are unlikely to succeed.

METASTASES

One of the hallmarks of cancer is its ability to spread, or metastasise, from one part of the body to another. The site in which a cancer originates is known as its primary site and the area to which it spreads is a secondary site. We have seen that tumours can cause problems by directly invading surrounding tissues. Cells from tumours can also spread through the blood-stream. Another route for cancer cells are the lymphatics, small channels running between the lymph glands which form part of the body's immune system. When tumour cells deposit in a lymph node it swells, much as the lymph nodes in your neck swell if you have a throat infection. The tumour can then travel from one lymph gland to the next by the lymphatic channels.

Not all cells in a cancer are capable of spreading to distant sites. Every time a cancer cell divides, though, it becomes more likely that at least one group, or clone, of daughter cells will have the ability to metastasise. This ability is thought to be under the control of genes, which either promote or suppress the ability to metastasise. As a cancer grows larger it becomes more likely that it will have spread beyond its primary site. In fact, at the time of treating a primary cancer, 60 per cent of patients will have either clinically apparent metastases or micro-scopic spread, which will eventually declare itself. Even when tumour cells reach the bloodstream, where they are very difficult to detect, there is no certainty that they will result in metastases. It appears that not only do you need the right type of cells to 'seed' other sites but they need to find the right 'soil' in which to grow.

The same type of primary tumour can metastasise to differ-ent organs. Fortunately, there are common patterns of spread for various tumours. Breast cancers, for example, most often spread to the liver, bones and lung. These organs are specifically targeted when we are searching clinically to find if a breast cancer has spread. Incidentally, when breast cancer spreads to the liver it should not be called liver cancer. Some patients become confused by this. It should still be called breast cancer because, under a microscope, it looks like the breast cancer tissue from which it came, not like liver cells, and will respond to drugs aimed at breast cancer. We discuss this later.

Much current research is directed at discovering how cancer cells spread and invade other organs. To spread, cancer cells must be able to break through the basement membrane, a barrier which separates the tissue where the cells originate from adjacent tissues. The supporting tissue between cells (called the extracellular matrix) and the basement membrane contain structural proteins. An example is collagen. Collagen fibres are like scaffolds which provide structure and strength to tissues. The collagen in basement membranes forms a lattice which incorporates another protein called laminin and all are coated with a third protein known as fibronectin.

The first thing a tumour cell must do before it can break out is detach itself from other tumour cells or cells of the body. Even this step is subject to regulation since there are proteins on the surface of cells, called cadherins, which determine how adhesive the cancer cells are to neighbouring cells. If there are numerous cadherins on the cell's surface, the tumour is less invasive. Alternatively, if the production of cadherins is lessened the tumour becomes more invasive.

Once free, the tumour cell attaches itself to the basement membrane. The proteins, laminin and fibronectin, facilitate this by binding to receptors on the surface of the cancer cells. Again, this binding can be pictured as keys being inserted into locks. After the cancer cell attaches to the basement membrane it must produce proteins, called enzymes, which digest the membrane and then clear a small area of the extracellular matrix so that the cell can penetrate it. This process is also subject to strict controls. It may be resisted by producing inhibitors of the digestive enzymes or simply by manufacturing more of the structural protein, collagen.

Let us say that the tumour cell has overcome the obstacles and broken through the basement membrane. If the invasion is going to be successful, the cancer cell must now be able to move into the destroyed matrix and find where to go next. Some cells, for example, will need to move across the matrix to enter blood vessels if they are to be spread via the bloodstream. At their destination, they will need to be able to move out again through the basement membrane of the blood vessels into the organ that is their new secondary site.

How cancer cells move

Studies of how cancer cells move have shown that there are many chemicals dissolved in the tissues that can attract cancer cells. Some are produced because of interactions between the host tissue and the cancer cell. These factors would explain how cancer cells know in which direction to move. However, unless cancer cells could move only in short bursts that depended on the local concentrations of these chemicals, other mechanisms for the movement must exist. The answer to this problem is that malignant cells have the ability to produce their own chemicals that stimulate their own motility, the so-called autocrine motility factors. These allow the cancer cell to move independently of the host tissues.

Observations of cancer cells show that, to move, they send out leg-like protrusions, or pseudopodia, into the surrounding tissues. These pseudopodia are responsible for finding the attracting chemicals in the surrounding tissue. They contain high concentrations of receptors for the matrix proteins so that they can attach to those proteins, just as the cancer cell initially attaches to the laminin and fibronectin of the basement membrane. Part of the movement of the cell, then, could be by a series of attaching and letting go of the surrounding tissues, propelling it along. It would be useful if the pseudopodia also contained some of the enzymes to dissolve the matrix to allow the cell to move through it.

Entering the secondary site

When circulating tumour cells reach their target organ they either stick to the lining cells of a small blood vessel in that organ or a clump of cells becomes wedged in the vessel. The cancer cells then attach to the basement membrane beneath the lining cells and the cells seal them off from the bloodstream. What follows is a process similar to that at the beginning, where the cancer must dissolve the basement membrane and move into its new home.

Angiogenesis

The formation of new blood vessels, a process known as angiogenesis, is necessary to transport food to both the primary and secondary cancer colony. Without blood vessels to supply nutrients to the cancer cells the cancer's growth could not extend beyond 2 millimetres, and growth in three dimensions would be difficult. Cancers can cause the growth of new blood vessels by producing chemicals which dissolve in the matrix around the cancer. This causes cells from the lining of very small blood vessels in the body to migrate out towards the tumour and sprout loops which grow into the cancer tissue. The way these blood vessel cells escape from the parent blood vessels and move into the matrix, dissolving it as they migrate, is very similar to the process described for cancer cells. It also has similar checks and balances. Factors have been found that promote the process and other factors that block it.

These new blood vessels not only carry nutrients for the cancer cells but also provide them with another handy path by which to escape and rapidly reach the bloodstream so they can spread throughout the body. The same process occurs at the other end of the cancer cell's journey when it is trying to colonise the organ where it has formed a secondary deposit. If the cancer grows too fast for this new blood supply, only the outer rim of the cancer will have nutrients and the centre breaks down.

Whether a cancer will grow in its new home depends on a balance between those factors produced by the cell and surrounding tissues which stimulate growth and those which inhibit it. Sometimes cancer cells can remain dormant for years, but are able to reactivate. The mechanisms for this are not well understood but the cells seem to be protected from the body's defences. Maybe the cells are not truly dormant, but the failure of growth beyond a very small size is due to the tumour's inability to form new blood vessels.

WHY IS RESEARCH INTO HOW CANCERS SPREAD SO USEFUL?

Piecing together the story of how cancers spread is not just interesting research. It has future applications in finding new anti-cancer treatments. Right now, it can help with predicting the likely outcome, or prognosis, for a patient with cancer.

As an example, the aggressiveness of an individual tumour can be predicted by the measurement of genes, or products of genes, that are associated with the process of invasion and spreading described above. A cell where there are genes producing products involved in metastasising is likely to be more aggressive than one without. It would also be worth finding what proportion of a tumour's cells has the ability to spread using probes for the markers associated with metastases. Some of the chemicals that we found to be associated with invasion may accumulate in the bloodstream and be measured there.

Many anti-cancer treatments are targeted at damaging the cell's DNA, thereby stopping the cell dividing (see Chapter 5). Now, whereas there may be a greater percentage of a tumour's cells in the growth phase when compared with the normal body's tissues, both divide by the same mechanism and both normal and cancer cells will be affected by the treatment. The ability to metastasise, however, sets a tumour apart from normal tissue. If we could target a treatment at some of the cascade of events that occur during the spread of cancers, we could expect better selectivity, sparing the normal tissues. This is where research into the mechanisms of metastasising holds such great promise for future treatments.

Anti-angiogenesis factors are already being tested. These may also stop tumour invasion since some of the mechanisms of the two are shared. Certainly, if new blood vessels cannot form, the size of the cancer is limited and the potential for spread beyond the primary site lessened.

Gene therapy, particularly inserting a gene to replace the function of a gene whose deletion is important in triggering the metastatic process, offers another possibility for treatment. Several of these approaches could be combined to help keep cancer cells under control.

DISTANT EFFECTS OF TUMOURS

A final testimony to the destructive power of cancer comes in considering the remote effects of cancer that are not due to the bulk of the primary or to its distant metastases. These so-called paraneoplastic syndromes arise because the tumour produces hormones, growth factors or other proteins which circulate round the body and affect other organs. Another mechanism for a distant effect arises when the body's immune system produces antibodies against the tumour and then these also react with normal tissues.

Although these distant effects are rare, the most common is when a tumour produces a hormone similar to the hormones produced by the normal glands in the body, but outside the normal controls and feedback mechanisms which regulate that hormone's production. For example, parathyroid hormone is secreted to help maintain the concentration of calcium in the bloodstream. If a tumour such as lung cancer overproduces a parathyroid-like hormone, the blood calcium will become too high and cause symptoms and signs in addition to those caused by the primary tumour and its metastases.

Often the abnormal production of the hormone will parallel the growth of the tumour and will be controlled by successful anti-cancer treatment. The symptoms of overproduction of a hormone may then reverse, but if the target organ is the kidney or nerve tissue, the reversibility of the effect will depend on the ability of the organ to repair the damage done to it.

CANCER RESEARCH

Most of the information that we have about the nature of cancer and its causes comes from research or observation. Basic research is done in the laboratory and seeks to explore the nature of cancer and how it grows and spreads using cancer cells and cancers in animals. Research into how to treat cancer begins in the laboratory by testing drugs and other substances for their ability to kill cancer cells. Eventually these results must be translated into the clinic to have an impact on the management of patients with cancer. This is when clinical trials are conducted.

Clinical trials are experiments which are planned in advance and follow a written protocol or plan. Most commonly they seek to test the effectiveness of a new treatment in patients with cancer. The initial trials of a new drug, called phase I trials, simply aim to establish a dose at which the drug can be given safely. The next trials, phase II trials, seek to establish the activity of the drug in shrinking various cancers. If a new treatment proves effective it must then be compared to the currently used treatment in a phase III trial. The endpoints of such a trial include the response of the tumour and the survival of the patient.

When conducting a clinical trial, the population or group of patients who is to participate must be defined. For example, decisions are made about what tumour types to test, the extent of disease which must be treated and how fit the patients must be to enter the trial. The extent of prior treatment may be a factor in selection of patients for a trial, since with each successive treatment the chances of responding become less. Also, patients should not participate in an experiment if an effective treatment exists. The established treatment should be used first and the experimental treatment tried subsequently.

Many of the design issues and language of clinical trials can be illustrated by the phase III trial. You can only do a phase III trial if there are two treatments which are effective but you don't know which is better. The idea of such a trial is to select two groups of patients to have the old or the new treatment so that they are matched in every characteristic except for the treatment they receive. Any differences between the two groups as they are followed up will then be due to the treatment. The group of patients receiving the standard treatment, called the control group, are there so that the group receiving the new treatment can be compared to them.

The researcher asks the statisticians how many patients will need to be entered into the trial to detect a difference between the two groups that would be clinically meaningful. For example a 20 per cent difference between treatments may be important but a 1 per cent difference may not.

Patients are randomly allocated to the two groups so that chance will take care of balancing the patient characteristics evenly. To ensure that there is no bias on the part of the patients or doctors, the trial can be designed so that neither knows which treatment they have been allocated, a process called blinding.

After the treatment, the patients in the two groups are followed by being seen in clinic regularly so that the response of the disease to the treatments and the survival of each group can be compared.

Clinical trials are suitable for assessing treatments when patients have cancer, but not for trying to answer questions like whether exposure to a particular substance or agent, such as asbestos, causes cancer. You can't randomise people to be exposed to asbestos or not. In this case, a group of people who are known to have been exposed to the agent in question can be matched to another group or cohort of the population who have identical characteristics except for the exposure to the agent being studied. The people in the two groups are then followed to see how many of each group develop cancer. This is called a cohort study and takes a long time. To try to get at the answer more quickly, patients with cancer can be matched with people without cancer and then their histories of exposure to the agent in question examined for differences. This is called a case-controlled study, where the people without cancer act as the control group much like the people having standard therapy were the control group for the patients receiving the experimental treatment.

These trials give us information about groups of people which we can then use to advise each individual patient.

SUMMARY

Cancer is the uncontrolled growth of cells and can arise in any part of the body. The loss of control has its basis in the genetic code in the nucleus of the cell. There can be mutations in genes which trigger cancer. Cancer promoting genes can be switched on and tumour suppressor genes switched off, allowing the cell to escape the control of signals from the rest of the body. The hallmark of cancer is the ability to invade tissues locally and spread to distant sites.

Now that we have explored the nature of cancer we can discuss its causes.

2

What causes cancer?

Every day when he looked into the glass, and gave the
last touch to his consummate toilette, he offered his
grateful thanks to Providence that his family was not
unworthy of him.

—*Benjamin Disraeli, Earl of Beaconsfield
1804–81, Lothair, Chap. I*

Is it genetic? This is a question often asked by patients with
cancer who are concerned about whether their children will
develop the same cancer. It may well have been asked by
Napoleon Bonaparte who was said to have died of stomach
cancer just as his father and grandfather had before him. What
they really want to know is whether the cancer can be inherited.
This is quite a different question. As we discovered in the
previous chapter, all cancers result from alterations to genes.
However, only a very small number of these alterations can be
inherited from our parents. For this to occur, the gene that is
altered must be in the reproductive or germ cells, which can
be passed on to the next generation, rather than in the somatic
cells (i.e. the cells of the rest of the body).

Most of the other alterations, or mutations as they are called,
result from a series of changes over the life of the somatic cells
and occur at the time that DNA is copied. Although there are

good mechanisms for making sure that DNA is copied accurately and there is the ability to correct mistakes, it is calculated that the division of any cell is associated with six new mistakes in the DNA sequence. This is not altogether a bad thing since it allows us a diversity in facing our changing environment, but it can also contribute to the development of cancer. Some mutations occur when cells are exposed to radiation, viruses or chemicals in the environment. The change is confined to those cells as they multiply during the lifetime of the individual. The two processes may overlap when, for example, you inherit a mutation which then makes you more susceptible to a factor in the environment which causes further mutations that result in cancer. The multi-step process of developing cancer is known as carcinogenesis and it is important to realise, when thinking about the causes of cancer, that we are not looking at a sudden event that immediately triggers cancer, but a process.

In this chapter we explore the process of carcinogenesis. We need to consider everything, from what we eat to what we are exposed to at work and in our environment, that could contribute to the development of cancer. The importance of discovering the factors that trigger cancer is that we may learn how to lessen our chances of developing cancer by changing our lifestyle.

You can't choose your parents, however, so first we explore some of the inherited cancers—that is, those that run in families.

CANCERS IN FAMILIES

As you know, genes come in pairs and we inherit one copy from each of our parents. There can be many forms of the one gene. Sometimes, one form of a gene will be dominant—when it is inherited from one parent the characteristic that it codes for will override that associated with the gene from the other parent. In this pattern of inheritance, if one parent with cancer carries a dominant form of the gene responsible, then the chance of the children inheriting the gene is 50 per cent. A child who inherits the dominant gene should have 100 per cent chance of developing the cancer. In fact, it is slightly less than that because the mutated gene doesn't always produce the cancer. Although there may be dominant susceptibilities to many types of cancer, they are rare, probably contributing to less than 5 per cent of cancers.

Other altered forms of genes that are inherited are only expressed if the same gene comes from both parents, or if a normal copy from one parent becomes altered or lost. These are recessive genes; inheriting one means that an individual is halfway to developing a disease but needs a further event that alters or knocks out the other gene of the pair before the disease can occur. Just carrying the gene, however, means the individual can pass it on to the next generation. In diseases associated with recessive genes, if both parents carry one altered form of the gene they will not have the disease, but each child has a one-in-four chance of inheriting both altered genes and thus the disease. The children have a one-in-four chance of inheriting both normal forms of the gene, and a two-in-four chance of inheriting one of each gene. In the latter case, they will not have the disease but are able to pass on the altered gene and are susceptible to developing the disease if something happens to their normal copy of the gene. Figure 2.1 gives some examples of these inheritance patterns as they apply to cancer.

A rare inherited childhood cancer

Retinoblastoma is a rare childhood cancer of the eye. It has been known to occur in families. Approximately four in ten of children with retinoblastoma inherited a dominant gene for this cancer. The retinoblastoma that occurs in families has different characteristics from the type that occurs sporadically. For example, it is more likely to affect both eyes. In the inherited form of the disease, it seems that two mutations in genes must occur. The first is a mutation in the retinoblastoma gene on one of the chromosomes in the germ cells that are inherited. Retinoblastoma develops if there is a further mutation in the

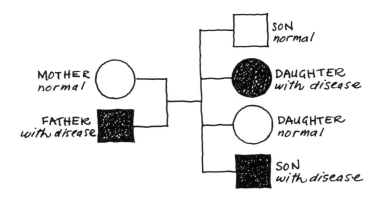

DOMINANT GENETIC DISORDER

One parent has a dominant gene for the disease.
Each child has a 50% chance of inheriting the disease.

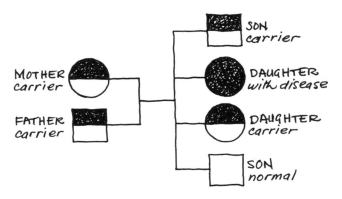

RECESSIVE GENETIC DISORDER

Both parents carry the gene but are free of the disease.
Each child has a 1 in 4 chance of inheriting both
abnormal genes and developing the disease and a
2 in 4 chance of inheriting one normal and one
abnormal gene and being a carrier.

Figure 2.1 Patterns of inheritance

second gene in the somatic cell. Furthermore, inheriting a susceptibility to retinoblastoma also makes the person more susceptible to other cancers, particularly the second cancers that can occur years after exposure to radiotherapy or chemotherapy.

A rare inherited bowel cancer

The susceptibility to cancer of the bowel can be dominantly inherited, although this is rare. The best known inherited bowel cancer is familial polyposis coli where affected individuals develop hundreds, if not thousands, of polyps (outgrowths from the lining of the bowel) in the large bowel wall by the time they are teenagers. If not treated, almost all these people will develop bowel cancer. The treatment to prevent them developing bowel cancer seems rather extreme. It involves removal of the whole of the large bowel before the cancers have a chance to develop. There is at present no other preventive measure.

The gene responsible for polyposis coli was eventually discovered on the fifth chromosome. Now called the APC gene, it is also found to be mutated in many sporadic cases of large bowel cancer. Most of the mutations in sporadic cancer result in inactivation of this gene. This makes a case for it being a tumour suppressor gene, since inactivation would then allow a cancer to develop.

Family cancer syndrome

In 1969, Frederick Li and Joseph Fraumeni described a group of families who had more than their fair share of cancers. Individuals in these families were susceptible to developing a range of cancers including breast cancers, sarcomas, bone cancers, brain tumours and leukaemias, among others. Family members were also susceptible to multiple cancers. Observations suggested that this propensity to cancer was inherited and, in 1990, mutations in a gene called p53 were found to be responsible for the family cancer syndrome, which now carries the names of the original observers, Li–Fraumeni.

More than 90 per cent of those who carry the mutated gene will develop cancer in their lifetime, with a 50 per cent chance of developing cancer by the age of 30. This compares with a 1 per cent chance of developing cancer by the age of 30 in the normal population and highlights one feature of inherited cancers—they occur in younger people.

The p53 gene is known to be a tumour suppressor gene. It had been known that alterations in the p53 gene could be associated with sporadic cancers. Now it has been found that some abnormalities in p53 could be inherited, since in the Li–Fraumeni syndrome the mutation was found in each cell, not just in the cancerous cells. Moreover, if an individual had only one normal copy of the p53 gene, he would be expected to be more cancer-prone since he requires only a further alteration in the one remaining copy.

This type of research, which identifies carriers of an abnormal gene, may alert people to be more rigorous with screening. In future, it is hoped that more can be done to prevent cancers when gene mutation carriers are identified. Investigating the mechanisms that enable genes to prevent cancer may allow the development of new therapeutic approaches.

Inheriting the susceptibility to breast cancer

The conditions discussed above are rare. It is more exciting to tell the story of the discovery of genes that increase the susceptibility to a common cancer such as breast cancer. Breast cancer will affect one in fourteen women, but it may be as few as 5 per cent who inherit a gene mutation that makes them more susceptible to it.

It was first reported in 1936 that breast cancer tended to cluster in families. A woman's increased risk of developing breast cancer depended on whether close, first-degree relatives such as mother or sisters had the disease, how many were affected and how young they were when they developed breast cancer. For example, if you have one close relative who developed breast cancer when she was over 50 years of age, your risk of developing the disease rises to one in eight. If you have two or more first-degree relatives who developed breast cancer when they were under 40 years old, your risk may approach one in two.

In 1990 Mary-Claire King and her team at the University of California reported that a gene that makes women susceptible to breast cancer may reside on chromosome seventeen. This gene was subsequently isolated and given the accurate, if unimaginative, name of BRCA 1. Indeed, it is one of the genes that, when altered, are associated with a susceptibility to breast cancer. Another gene that increases susceptibility to breast cancer, BRCA 2, has been found on chromosome thirteen. Yet another is the p53 gene that we discussed in relation to the family cancer syndrome. All these genes behave as if they are tumour suppressor genes, since the loss of the normal gene results in cancer.

The normal function of BRCA 1 when unaltered is unknown. When it is altered it accounts for about half the inherited susceptibilities to breast cancer. For BRCA 1 to cause breast cancer, both copies of the gene must be either lost or mutated. Several different mutations have been recorded. For example, one specific mutation of particular interest (called 185delAG) has been discovered in families of Ashkenazi Jewish background.

Women who have inherited one abnormal copy of BRCA 1 need only a few more damaging mutations in their lifetime to develop cancer. However, BRCA 1, unlike p53, has not been associated with somatic mutations that cause sporadic breast cancer. Children of parents with a mutation in one of their BRCA 1 genes have a 50 per cent chance of inheriting the 'bad' gene.

Women who carry a mutated BRCA 1 gene have a 90 per cent risk of developing cancer, with half the cases occurring by the age of 50 and 85 per cent by the age of 70. Again, inherited forms of breast cancer are more likely to occur in younger women, with one in four breast cancers in women younger than 30 involving inherited susceptibilities. Women who inherit a mutated BRCA 1 gene also have an increased risk of developing ovarian cancer. An increased risk of developing cancer of the large bowel has also been reported.

Men who inherit a mutated BRCA 1 do not appear to have the same increased risk of developing breast cancer, but may have an increased susceptibility to prostate cancer. If men inherit mutations in BRCA 2, however, this is associated with an increased risk of breast cancer.

Testing for genetic mutations is discussed, with screening, in Chapter 4. Many issues are involved since the result affects not only the individual tested but the whole family.

Inherited cancers

The search for cancer-causing genes is well under way in other cancers and many more will be discovered as more genes of our DNA are identified. Even in common tumours, inherited susceptibilities are rare, as illustrated by using the results of the research into familial breast cancer. We should therefore explore the factors in our environment that can cause mutations in the genes of the rest of the somatic cells. First, though, I would like to highlight the multi-step process needed to develop a cancer, the process of carcinogenesis.

THE PROCESS OF DEVELOPING CANCER

It is important to stress that the development of cancer is not a sudden event. It is a chain of events over a period of time. As we have seen, the step that starts the ball rolling may be a mutation in a single cell. This could have been inherited or caused by something in the environment. At this stage the cell is not cancerous but the process has been initiated. The next step is for a cancer-causing agent to persuade the precancerous cells to divide to form a group of cells. Again, this expansion of the mutated cells does not result in cancer. It results in precancerous lumps, such as polyps in the bowel, which become larger and more abnormal. The agents that promote this change may be viruses or chemicals or even agents from the body, such as hormones, which can promote breast or prostate cancer. The cells where the cancer process has been initiated respond differently to the cancer-promoting agents from the way normal cells would, and so the initiated cells are selected to grow.

The precancerous clump of cells often becomes cancerous without the need for additional outside influences if further changes occur to the cells' genes, such as their loss during further cell divisions. If, however, the precancerous cells are exposed again to tumour-promoting agents, the change to cancer is accelerated by inflicting further damage on the genes of the precancerous cells.

The process of triggering a cell to become cancerous, then promoting its growth into a precancerous lump, which after further genetic change becomes cancerous, can take a long time. Even if damage to the DNA is caused by cancer-promoting agents in the environment, the cell can sometimes repair the damage before a cancer results.

People often wonder why they developed cancer when the next-door neighbour didn't. By understanding the process that causes cancer, we can now reply that it is a combination of genetic susceptibility, mistakes made during copying of the DNA and environmental stimuli, all of which have to affect the cells over time. If you have the susceptibility but there is nothing to promote growth of the abnormal cells, then no cancer occurs. If you don't have the susceptibility, then exposure to known cancer-causing agents like cigarette smoke may not trigger cancer. We can also see now why you will not be able to pick the day the cancer started or the event that caused it.

CANCER AND THE ENVIRONMENT

How do we discover which agents in our environment increase our risk of developing cancer? In the scientific world we look for experimental evidence. Sometimes we know that a particular chemical or hormone causes cancer in animals. This can be useful, but cannot always be directly related to humans.

We can look for reports in the scientific literature of cases of unusual associations between exposure to a particular substance and the later development of cancer. We are all exposed to so many substances in our environment that isolating one can be difficult. Determining whether a substance is causative is easier if exposure is confined to a selected group and the tumour is otherwise uncommon. An example is the association between asbestos exposure and the development of mesothelioma, a rare cancer of the outer lining of the lungs. When many cases of this rare tumour began appearing in individuals who shared in common only the fact that they had worked in an asbestos mine, or in the building trade where asbestos was used for insulation, then the identification of asbestos as a cause for the cancer was possible. Imagine how difficult it could be to prove, say, that motor car exhaust gases cause cancer, since most of us are exposed regularly to these pollutants.

Epidemiologists study populations (selected groups of people) to discover such statistically important associations between factors in our environment and cancer. If they want to investigate whether exposure to a particular substance causes cancer, they follow (monitor) a group of people who have been exposed and find another group of people who are matched in every other respect except for the exposure and see if cancer occurs more frequently in the exposed group.

There are some general characteristics that are well established. Most cancers are more common in older age groups. Any deviation from this general rule requires an explanation. For example, the lessening rate of increase of breast cancer following menopause suggests that the female hormones, oestrogens, may have an important impact on the cause of the disease.

Most cancers are more common in men. The increasing incidence of lung cancer in men in the first half of this century may relate to their greater smoking habits at this time. Over the last few decades, since women became liberated to smoke, their rate of lung cancer has been steadily increasing.

Differences have been found in cancer incidence between countries and even between different socioeconomic groups. Dietary patterns or occupational exposures of specific races or groups have been suggested to explain these differences.

Let us explore some of the factors in our environment that are linked to causing cancer. We will start with the best known, tobacco.

Smoking and cancer

Smoking is associated with three of every ten cancer deaths. Eight of every ten lung cancer deaths in men and just under that in women are due to smoking. Other cancers associated with smoking include cancers of the head and neck region, bladder, kidney and pancreatic cancers. Smoking has been implicated in leukaemia and in the development of polyps in the large bowel.

Although we tend to focus on smoking and cancer, just as deadly are the heart disease, airways disease and strokes which are more likely in tobacco smokers. It has been estimated that one in every four smokers dies as a result of smoking. Those who smoke more than twenty cigarettes every day reduce their lifespan by around fifteen years as compared with non-smokers.

The good news is that if you give up cigarette smoking there is a gradual fall in your risk of death from lung cancer. This does not happen immediately and the risk may be higher than for non-smokers for as long as 25 years. Giving up smoking at a younger age has more impact on reducing the risk of cancer than if you wait until you are older. The benefit in reducing the risk of heart disease becomes apparent more quickly, possibly by one year.

Smoking, unfortunately, does not impact only on the smoker. Probably two-thirds of the smoke from a cigarette goes into the atmosphere and can affect those around the smoker. So-called passive smoking has been more difficult to isolate as a risk factor for cancer. Certainly, breakdown products from tobacco smoke can be measured in the bodies of the partners of smokers. They may have about one-third higher risk of lung cancer than non-smokers.

Why does smoking cause cancer? Cigarette smoke contains chemical carcinogens. These chemicals can promote cancer by causing mutations in the cells' genes. Although we are talking here about environmental causes of cancer, there are inherited factors that determine whether a person can break down these cancer-causing chemicals. Indeed, some people can inherit the ability to activate these carcinogens. These chemicals will ultimately cause changes in the genes which may add to other inherited or acquired changes over time and eventually promote the development of cancer. Many gene mutations have been found to be associated with lung cancers. Whether cancer results from exposure to these carcinogens may depend on whether the cell can repair the damage in time. The rate of repair is another factor that can be inherited. Therefore, some people who smoke will be more prone to developing cancer than others, depending on what tendencies they have inherited. The fact that an individual lives a full life span despite smoking heavily is his good genetic fortune, rather than support for claims that cigarette smoking does not cause cancer.

There are other environmental factors such as drinking alcohol or being exposed to other cancer-causing substances at work which can add to the likelihood that a smoker will develop cancer. We will explore some of these factors.

Alcohol drinking and cancer

If you had to choose between vices in relation to cancer risk, smoking is by far the worst. It has been difficult to assess the effects of alcohol alone because the major risk seems to be in people who are both heavy drinkers and smokers. This combination is implicated in cancers in the head and neck area—the mouth, throat and oesophagus. Alcohol probably contributes to three in every hundred cancers. It is not certain how alcohol interacts with smoking to increase the risk of these cancers but reducing drinking to a more moderate degree decreases the risk.

It is well known that heavy alcohol drinking causes cirrhosis, or scarring of the liver. This in turn can result in primary cancers of the liver, which are otherwise rare in Western society. Alcohol itself can also increase the incidence of liver cancers.

There is speculation about alcohol drinking and other cancers. Breast cancer may be related to alcohol consumption, but it has been difficult to assess precisely the contribution of alcohol as opposed to other risk factors.

Cancer and the workplace

Medical students have grown up on the story of Percival Pott who, in 1775, suggested that chimney sweeps developed more than their fair share of cancer of the scrotum because of their exposure to soot as they swept the chimneys. This demonstrated not only that factors in the environment could cause cancer, but described the first cancer clearly related to occupation. It is particularly important to identify carcinogens in the workplace, since cancer can be prevented by reducing or eliminating the exposure of workers to these substances.

It can be very difficult to establish a link between exposure to a chemical at work and the later development of cancer, since the events will be separated by a long time. Sometimes, information on cancer hazards at work has come initially from multiple reports from the experience of doctors treating their individual patients. Other associations have been found in studies of large populations of people where the aim of the study was to look for cancer risk factors. Most of the definite links between exposure to a cancer-causing substance in the workplace and the subsequent development of cancer have occurred when a relatively rare cancer has been found in workers with a very specific exposure that would not occur in the general environment.

Asbestos and mesothelioma

A good example of the link between cancer and the workplace is the association between asbestos exposure and the development of mesothelioma, a rare cancer of the outer covering of the lung or lining of the abdomen. The Australian experience illustrates this. The incidence of mesothelioma in Australia has been steadily increasing, having trebled since 1980. Australia now has the highest rate of mesothelioma in the industrialised world, at just over nineteen cases for every million of population. This is due to past occupational exposure to asbestos. It can be 20 to 40 years between asbestos exposure and the development of mesothelioma. Seven of every 100 cases are related to occupational or environmental exposure at just one asbestos mining town, Wittenoom in Western Australia. Australian registry figures show that nearly three out of every four cases of mesothelioma have a past history of asbestos exposure.

Other occupations that are associated with asbestos exposure, and where workers are now developing mesothelioma, include the asbestos cement production industry and the insulation industry. Building and demolition workers and boilermakers, often from railway yards and shipyards, also had contact with asbestos.

Not all types of asbestos fibres are associated with the same risk of cancer. Fibres that are more needle-like, such as crocidolite, are more carcinogenic than the curly fibres such as chrysotile. This may be because the needle-like fibres are more likely to lodge in small airways where they stay for longer than the shorter or thicker fibres. Certainly, the number of fibres correlates with the likelihood of developing cancer. Asbestos fibres are thought to cause the deletion of parts of chromosomes, thus helping to cause cancer.

Mesothelioma is not the only type of cancer associated with asbestos exposure. There is also an increase in lung cancer. And if you smoke you have a greater risk of developing lung cancer after asbestos exposure.

Other occupations at risk of specific cancers

Many other occupational exposures have been linked with cancers. Sometimes the tumour is rare. Exposure to vinyl chloride in the manufacture of polyvinyl chloride can cause the uncommon tumour, angiosarcoma of the liver. Sometimes a tumour is common but seen more frequently in workers with specific jobs. Analine dye workers have a higher incidence of bladder cancer. Leather workers are prone to developing cancers of the nasal sinuses and bladder. Benzene, used in the petroleum industry, can predispose to the development of leukaemia. Exposure to arsenic used in mining and smelting increases the risk of developing lung and skin cancers. The exposure need not always be to an exotic chemical or a substance that sounds toxic. There is a surprising association between exposure to wood dust in hardwood furniture making and developing cancer in the nasal sinuses.

If we link genetic predispositions with occupational exposures, it is interesting to speculate whether people will be barred from certain occupations if their genetic risk of a particular cancer is high. We will know more about the function of genes in the body as a result of the human genome project which seeks to map every gene in the human cell. Individuals with certain genes could find themselves with high life insurance premiums!

Workers will also be at risk from exposures that affect us all. Outdoor jobs carry the risk of sun exposure and skin cancer. Smoking may be even more of a luxury if smokers are also exposed at their workplace to other carcinogens that cause lung cancer. Let us look at environmental factors that affect us all.

Diet and cancer

You are what you eat. This is an old saying which many of us hope is not accurate. Nonetheless, we are all aware that we can adversely affect our health by what we eat. The link between cholesterol and saturated fats and heart disease, for example, has been well publicised and is well supported by clinical trials in the medical journals.

There are also associations between certain foods and cancer. Some foods may be a factor in causing cancer and some may have a role in cancer prevention. Unlike the situations described above, it is much harder to show the relationship between food and common cancers, since eating is only one of a number of activities that form part of our lifestyle and contribute to our environmental exposure. As a result, there is some scientific uncertainty about the role of specific foods. Associations that are difficult to prove may also be difficult to definitely rule out. This allows for all manner of theories relating food to cancer and the bookshops are full of such speculation. You will find outrageous claims, such as curing all types of cancer by just altering what you eat.

Before outlining the current scientific facts on diet and cancer it may be helpful to list some points to consider when evaluating popular books on diet and cancer. First, the fact that a vitamin can be shown to alter cancer cells in a laboratory may not translate to what happens in the body. Second, foods that have the potential to *prevent* cancer should not be assumed to have any role in curing it once it has developed. Also, if too much of a food is bad for you, that does not mean it should be completely excluded from the diet. This could leave a gap in nutrition that could be harmful, particularly as the rest of the body needs to be as healthy as possible to fight cancer. And, equally, if a food is good for you, it does not follow that ten times as much is ten times as good. The body will just get rid of what it doesn't need. This is often the rationale of some unorthodox practitioners who advocate high doses of vitamins and other trace elements. When given in this way they are no longer natural products but drugs, where side effects must be balanced with any benefits. There is no doubt that the body prefers to take these nutrients as part of natural foods rather than as purified supplements. In general, a dietary supplement should only be required if your diet is poor, or you can't eat, and there is a deficiency in that nutrient.

Fat

Fat in the diet has been suggested as a risk factor, particularly for breast and bowel cancer. This was based on studies which showed that countries with a high fat intake per person also had these cancers occurring more often. It has been difficult to show a strong relationship between fat and breast cancer in studies where one group of people is matched to another in all characteristics, except for their fat intake, and the incidence of breast cancer compared in the two groups with different fat intakes. It has also been difficult to show any big impact of fat intake on the behaviour of breast cancer once it has developed. Another confounding factor is whether we are talking of poly-unsaturated or saturated fats. It seems that the polyunsaturated fats are more likely to be the culprits. A tantalising observation is that southern Europeans have a high intake of mono-unsaturated fats in the form of olive oil. Their cancer rates are less than other groups with similar or lower overall fat intakes.

Stronger associations have been shown between high fat intake and red meat consumption and the development of cancer of the large bowel. An overall analysis of thirteen studies, though, showed a relationship between overall calorie intake and bowel cancer but was not convincing that the relationship was specifically with fats. Even the association with meat may not be due to the fat content but other substances in meat.

Although less work has been done in prostate cancer, the consumption of animal fat correlates strongly with the death rate from prostate cancer. Again, the type of fat is important since there is no correlation with vegetable fats.

Fibre

In the 1970s, Burkitt made the observation that diseases such as large bowel cancer were common in Western countries where a lot of refined food was eaten and low in African nations where high-fibre diets were common. It was suggested that fibre protects against cancer of the large bowel. There are simple mechanisms by which this may occur. Fibre traps fluids which would dilute carcinogens in the bowel, or the amount of carcinogen produced may be decreased by the presence of the fibre. Fibre would also increase the bulk in the large bowel and decrease the transit time through the bowel. Dietary fibre may also be protective against breast cancer by decreasing the processing and re-uptake of oestrogens in the bowel. This may also apply to other hormone-sensitive tumours.

It is difficult to be absolutely certain of the role of fibre because fruit and vegetables, which are a major source of fibre, also contain other substances that may protect against cancer. These are often referred to as micronutrients and include vitamins and trace elements.

Micronutrients

The micronutrients from fruit and vegetables can help prevent cancer at all stages of its development. At the initiation stage, where DNA damage occurs, folate and B vitamins participate in DNA repair. Cancer promotion, which means producing greater numbers of the cell with the mutated DNA, can be slowed by agents that affect growth rates. These agents include vitamin A, retinoids and folate. Retinoids and antioxidants also inhibit growth in the progression of a tumour. It is difficult to demonstrate the cancer-preventive effects of micronutrients in fruit and vegetables because there is no way of telling when and if a cancer would have developed. Studies that monitor people until the development of cancer take many years to arrive at an answer. We return to the effect of specific micronutrients on specific cancers with the discussion of prevention in Chapter 8.

Cancer-causing agents in food

Food contaminants or additives, or even the way the food is prepared, may result in taking in carcinogens with the food. Aflatoxins produced by a fungus can contaminate peanuts or maize, resulting in a higher risk of liver cancer. Fish preserved by salting develops high concentrations of nitrosamines which are associated with causing nasopharyngeal cancer. Cooking practices, such as frying food in hot oil, may lead to the production of carcinogens which are then ingested with food.

Perhaps it is fortunate that there are also naturally occurring anti-carcinogens in food. Food, however, is only one aspect of our environment—we are exposed to many other factors.

Cancer and pollution

There are many unpleasant pollutants in our environment which we intuitively believe must be bad for us. This is particularly so in industrialised urban areas where we are concerned about pollution ranging from car exhausts and pesticides through to electromagnetic fields from powerlines. It has been difficult to study the impact of many of these pollutants, where the exposure is to multiple agents at low levels, when overwhelming causes of cancer, such as cigarette smoking, exist in the same environment.

It has been estimated that environmental pollution accounts for only two of every 100 cancers. The products from burning fossil fuels are suggested as causative factors in developing lung cancer. Certainly, hydrocarbons can produce characteristic gene mutations. However, precise figures on the increased risks associated with these factors in isolation are difficult to obtain.

Pesticides and herbicides cause cancer in laboratory animals at high doses and with long exposures to the agents. They do not directly alter genes. Again, it is difficult to determine the impact on the normal population, so researchers in the United States have studied farmers who should have higher levels of exposure. They were interested in farmers who had developed lymphomas and leukaemias to see if their exposure to pesticides was greater than other farmers. In summary, there is very little difference between farmers and the rest of the population. However, farmers who had used the herbicide 2,4 D (2,4 dichlorophenoxyacetic acid) for long periods were more prone to developing lymphomas.

A few studies have investigated the contamination of drinking water. Particular concern is with the products formed as a result of chlorination and their link with slightly increased risks of bladder cancer. Even if a low risk does exist, this must be

41

counterbalanced by the benefits of eliminating infectious agents from the water.

There has been great public interest in the relationship between developing cancer and exposure to the low-frequency electric and magnetic fields around electric power transmission lines. A study from Denver in the United States has suggested an increased risk in childhood cancer. Other studies are confusing because they have yielded both negative and positive results. The magnetic fields produced by powerlines are very weak and would not be expected to cause DNA damage. No study has been able to provide convincing evidence linking proximity to powerlines with adult cancers. The association between living near electric power transmission lines and developing cancer cannot be definitely ruled out, but neither has it been proven.

Some of the damage attributed to electromagnetic radiation as microwaves is due to the heat produced. Heat is not produced by the low-frequency fields generated from powerlines. Chronic exposure to heat can be a problem, however, as shown by cancers occurring in people who sit with their legs close to the fire for long periods. The same risk occurs with the use of warming pans or hot water bottles close to the skin over a long time, which may cause tissue damage. It may not be the heat alone that causes cancer but it may make it easier for other stimuli to do so.

We always think of environmental exposures as occurring mainly outside our homes. This is not the case. For example, some studies have linked cooking oil vapours or the products of coal fires to increased cancer risk. These may add to the risks from tobacco smoke in the home, or fibres or chemicals brought in on work clothes to the family laundry. Indoor air pollution with radon gas is another risk we should discuss.

RADIATION AND CANCER

When considering radiation we must look at ionising radiation (i.e. radiation with enough energy to knock electrons from atoms or molecules). This can come from natural sources, as with radon gas, from nuclear accidents and explosions, or from the diagnostic use of x-rays and ultraviolet radiation from the sun.

Ionising radiation

Unfortunately, we have learned much of what we know about the cancer caused by radiation exposure by monitoring survivors of the atomic bomb attacks on Hiroshima and Nagasaki. We know that the cancer occurs late. Leukaemias appear in five to seven years after the exposure, but solid tumours can occur over the rest of a lifetime. The likelihood of developing a solid tumour is increased if the exposure to the radiation occurs at a young age. The risk is slightly greater for women because breast tissue is particularly susceptible. The thyroid gland is another target but any other solid tumour can occur.

One of the first organs described as developing cancer after radiation exposure was the bones, when painters who painted the luminous dials on watches later developed bone cancer by ingesting radium-containing paint, through the habit of licking their paintbrushes into a point.

Radiation causes deletions and rearrangements in DNA. This may cause oncogenes to be activated or tumour suppressor genes to be inactivated.

Most of us will avoid radiation exposure from atomic bombs or nuclear power plant accidents but we can still be exposed to radiation in our homes. It has long been known that uranium miners are exposed to radon gas which is inhaled and adds to the risk of lung cancer. Radon is a naturally occurring gas which rises from the ground where there is a certain amount of uranium in the rock and soil. The radon level in a house will depend on where it is built but it can be assumed from the miners' experience that an increased risk of lung cancer will be seen in certain areas. In the United States it is estimated that up to 12 per cent of homes may be exposed to an unacceptably high level of radon.

The other major radiation exposure occurs when radiation is used to treat cancer or for diagnostic x-rays. Radiation therapy can cause late second cancers but is probably responsible for only a small percentage of them. Radiation most commonly produces cancers at the site of the radiation or leukaemias and the likelihood of doing so is related to the dose given. That is no reason, though, to limit the dose of radiation given and compromise the efficacy of the treatment of the first cancer, since the second cancer is a late effect which patients would only survive to develop if they were successfully treated for their initial malignancy. We do know that combining radiotherapy with chemotherapy increases the risk of second cancers and so we may be able to limit the situations when we have to do this.

Diagnostic x-rays are more of a problem—we don't want to expose people to great risks of cancer as part of diagnostic tests. This applies even more so if we are already using x-rays for screening, such as mammograms to screen for breast cancer. We know that x-ray workers developed skin cancers in the days before stringent safety standards were enforced. Now, the exposure from diagnostic x-rays is not in the same league as from radiation therapy so patients with cancer need not be concerned about additional exposure from diagnostic tests. Across the rest of the population, figures would suggest that an excess of cancers should occur due to diagnostic radiation exposure. When broken down to the risk to an individual, however, things are placed in perspective. The risk to an individual that the x-ray of a limb will cause death from cancer is one in two and a half million. Other procedures with multiple x-rays or CT scans will have a higher risk than that, but it will still be relatively small compared with the other cancer-causing factors we have discussed.

Screening mammograms deserve special mention. Here any risk of the procedure must be balanced against the benefits of the early detection of breast cancer. As women become older the chance of mammography reducing the risks of dying from breast cancer becomes greater and the risk of late mortality from breast cancer becomes less. It follows that the recommendation to screen women over 50 years (see Chapter 4) fits well in terms of the relative risk of the mammogram.

Sun exposure and cancer

Advertising campaigns such as 'Slip Slop Slap' (slip on a shirt, slop on some sunscreen and slap on a hat) have made most people aware of the risks of skin cancer with exposure to the ultraviolet rays of the sun. Greater exposure to ultraviolet radiation could be expected with depletion of the protective ozone layer in the upper atmosphere. Non-melanoma skin cancers are the commonest cancers in the world and are increasing. Melanoma skin cancers are particularly nasty—if they spread beyond the skin they have a high death rate. Prolonged exposure to the sun, such as may occur with outdoor occupations or sun-worshipping, is associated with the development of non-melanoma skin cancers. Ultraviolet rays damage DNA which eventually leads to the formation of a cancer. Melanomas result from intense exposure to the sun with episodes of acute sunburn. Exposure to ultraviolet rays not only damages DNA but also suppresses the immune system, which makes it easier for skin cancers to develop.

Skin cancer is far more common in white populations, particularly if they have migrated to latitudes with greater sun exposure. The melanin pigment in the skin protects darker-skinned people. Australian Aborigines, for example, develop melanomas only on depigmented areas such as the soles and palms or the lining of the mouth. There is a genetic predisposition to melanoma which makes it more likely in some individuals.

Another condition predisposing to skin cancer is the genetically inherited disease, xeroderma pigmentosum. This reduces the ability of cells to repair ultraviolet damage to DNA, thus increasing the risk of sun-related skin cancers.

INFECTIONS CAUSING CANCER

I start this section with a disclaimer. In general, most infections don't cause cancer and cancer is not contagious. I emphasise this because I have had to counsel patients whose grandchildren

45

were not allowed to hug them after they were diagnosed with cancer, in case they caught it. I have also seen couples who were scared of intimacy after one partner developed cancer. These misapprehensions are tragic, particularly as they occur at a time when the patient needs close human contact more than ever. There are specific situations, though, when the development of cancer is related to infectious agents.

Viruses and cancer

It was a cancer that alerted doctors to the emergence of a new disease, the acquired immunodeficiency syndrome (AIDS), and the eventual discovery of its viral aetiology in the 1980s. Until then, Kaposi's sarcoma had been an unusual slow-growing cancer confined to the legs of elderly Mediterranean or Jewish men. When it began appearing in a much more aggressive form over the bodies and on the linings of the mouth, stomach and bowels of young homosexual men, it was clear that something unusual was happening. This unusual happening was the suppression of the men's immune system. The cause was later discovered to be a virus, the human immunodeficiency virus (HIV).

Kaposi's sarcoma is not the only cancer associated with HIV infection. Lymphomas occur, tending to be more aggressive than their counterparts without HIV infection. They occur more often in organs, particularly the brain, rather than predominating in lymph glands. These cancers have always been associated with a depressed immune state.

Cancer of the cervix in women, often secondary to papilloma virus infection, shares with HIV infection the fact that they are both sexually transmitted. There is a very high chance of Pap smear tests being abnormal in HIV-positive women. There is also a high prevalence of HIV positivity in young women diagnosed with cancer of the cervix. The tumours tend to be more aggressive when associated with AIDS.

Let us move now to another virus-related cancer. Although uncommon in the West, cancer of the liver is frequent in

South-East Asia. In the 1970s it was observed that the distribution of cases of liver cancer was the same as the distribution of cases of hepatitis B virus. In fact, chronic infection with the hepatitis B virus has been associated with a risk of developing liver cancer 100 times greater than people who are not infected. The virus may cause cancer in two ways. It may stimulate cell growth in response to liver cell injury or its DNA may enter a cell.

The final virus we discuss is the Ebstein-Barr virus (EBV), known for causing glandular fever. Cancer arises in cells infected with this virus. The virus can alter genes as one step on the road to cancer. In Africa, the virus is associated with a very aggressive form of lymphoma, Burkitt's lymphoma, which has a very rapid doubling time. Burkitt's lymphoma, due to EBV, occurs usually in association with the effects on the immune system of the widespread malaria found in Africa. In other places EBV is involved with lymphomas which occur in immune deficiency diseases.

Bacteria

Helicobacter pylori is a bacterium which can be isolated from people with inflammation of the stomach, whether they have symptoms or not. An association of this organism with stomach cancer has been found in patients with high levels of antibodies to helicobacter. There is a long time between infection and the development of cancer. Lymphoma of the stomach is also associated with this infection. Antibiotics to eradicate the bacteria are now used with anti-cancer agents to cure these tumours. It seems likely that helicobacter pylori is a contributing factor to developing cancer but requires other factors to come into play.

Parasites

Included for completeness is the association between the bladder parasite, Schistosoma haemotobium, and the development of the uncommon squamous cell cancer of the bladder. The parasite is thought to enhance the formation of cancer-causing N-nitroso compounds. It is common in the developing world.

HORMONES AND CANCER

It has been suggested that hormones can be associated with cancer by overstimulation of organs that are responsive to hormones. After a gene mutation has occurred, the hormones may drive the cells to divide and allow the development of the cancerous cell population. In breast cancer, anything that causes greater exposure of the breast to hormones increases the risk of cancer. Therefore, early onset of menses, late menopause and hormone replacement therapy are risk factors. Early pregnancies tend to be protective because, although they increase hormone levels early on, they reduce the free hormone levels in the longer term. Breast feeding, by delaying the return of menstrual cycles, is also a protective factor. Obesity, on the other hand, is associated with an increase in female hormone levels and is thus a risk factor.

Similar comments apply to endometrial cancer (i.e. cancer of the lining of the uterus) and ovarian cancer. Additional hormones are now given to women as part of oral contraception or hormone replacement therapy around the time of the menopause. These treatments may carry the risk of promoting cancer.

MEDICATIONS AND CANCER

Unfortunately, the cause of some cancers has been traced back to medication prescribed for another condition. To use a hormonal example, synthetic oestrogens given to women during pregnancy were found to cause cancers of the vagina and cervix in their daughters several years later. There is certainly a concern about the risk of endometrial cancer in patients taking hormone replacement therapy, and of breast cancer after prolonged use of oral contraceptives.

Anti-cancer chemotherapy drugs, particularly a class of drugs called alkylating agents, have been found to cause second cancers a few years after they are given. Leukaemias and lymphomas are common second cancers. Again, there is no value in compromising the treatment of the initial cancer to eliminate this risk, but the risk of second cancers must be weighed against the benefits. Different drug combinations without alkylating agents need to be developed to lessen this late side effect.

Not all medications may be harmful. There have been reports that aspirin, for example, which is used as an anti-inflamatory agent may protect against large bowel cancer.

STRESS AND CANCER

There is much speculation about the role of stress in causing cancer. Many therapies aimed at relieving stress have been advocated as treatments for cancer. There is a complex relationship between psychological states and physical wellbeing. Stress may be able to change the immune system and hormone levels. It has been difficult, though, to establish stress as a cause of cancer, independent of other causes. A reason for this may be illustrated by simply stating that increased stress may be associated with increased smoking, overeating or becoming 'run down', all of which may impact on the development of cancer.

Intuitively, we may question the strength of the association between stress and cancer because we all know people who lead high-stress lives and don't develop cancer, and layabouts who do. I also have a problem with doctors who tell patients that their stressful lifestyle caused their cancer. This adds to the burden that patients must bear since they blame themselves for developing cancer, when it is not the case. Stress can be a nice intangible explanation but adds to the burden of the diagnosis.

Intuition is not very scientific, so what do the studies show? Well, for a start, it has proved difficult to define stress, since the concept varies between individuals. What many of the studies have done is to look at social stress factors, such as the death of a loved one or examinations. Several studies have suggested an increased death rate in people who have recently lost a relative. This includes cancer deaths, but a recent bereavement can't have been the cause of the cancer since, as we have seen, the cancer probably started developing years before.

Many studies have focused on breast cancer risk. One large National Cancer Institute study in the United States showed no association between stressful life events and the risk of breast cancer. Other studies, however, have linked stressful life events to the recurrence of breast cancer and yet others have suggested an increased incidence of breast cancer in highly stressed individuals.

Spiegel has claimed that regular psychological support improves survival in cancer patients. We await other studies to see if the improvement in survival was due to the psychological support or related to other factors, such as other treatments used. Certainly, Greer and others have reported that patients who respond to the diagnosis of cancer with a fighting spirit do better than more passive individuals.

Much more needs to be learned about psychological factors in the aetiology of cancer but, until we have such facts, definite statements about the relationship between stress and cancer should not be made.

SUMMARY

Cancer is caused by mutations in the genes of cells. Several events need to occur over a period of time. There are events that initiate cancer and others that promote it. Some of the changes in genes can be inherited from our parents. This places us at greater risk of developing cancer because it will take fewer acquired changes in the genes to trigger cancer. Many factors in our environment, including smoking, what we eat and what we are exposed to at work and in our homes, can combine to make a group of cells become malignant.

3

How do you diagnose cancer?

. . . seek, and ye shall find.

—The Holy Bible, *King James Version, Matthew 7.7*

'The definitive test for cancer is a biopsy'—this is what I keep telling medical students to encourage them to do a biopsy first rather than a thousand other tests. What I mean is this: if you can feel a lump or see it on an x-ray or scan, you should take a piece of it, the biopsy, as soon as possible and have a pathologist look at it under a microscope to tell you what it is. Other tests may then help you to decide how widespread the tumour is and what bodily functions it is disrupting. There are many ways of getting at a tumour. There are many tests that the pathologist can do to find out what the tumour is. There are many different types of scans and x-rays to help find the tumour in the first place. In this chapter we discuss how all these come together to help diagnose cancer.

HOW TO BIOPSY A TUMOUR

Samples of tissue can be obtained in many different ways. Major advances in this area have made life so much easier for patients.

For example, we now have simple procedures for obtaining tissue samples instead of needing an open operation. Thin needles can be accurately inserted into lumps in the chest or abdomen using scans to guide the needles. Previously, an open surgical biopsy was required but now this is only needed if the other methods fail or a larger piece of tumour is required to make a diagnosis.

Flexible endoscopes, which by means of optic fibres and lights allow their users to see into passages of the body, such as the bowels or air passages, also allow the operator to perform biopsies of any abnormal tissue that is seen. Examples of tissue which may be sampled in this way are polyps in the bowel or tumours growing in the walls of airways. Lumps pressing from the outside on an air passage can also be biopsied by a needle which is guided from the endoscope through the wall of the airway into the tissue beside it, again avoiding more invasive surgery. Similarly, rigid instruments called laparoscopes can be used to look into the chest or abdominal cavities and need only a small puncture wound rather than a surgical cut to reach their target.

The second major advance, which goes hand in hand with simpler procedures, is the ability to make a diagnosis of cancer on smaller and smaller pieces of tissue. Cytology is about making a diagnosis from single cells. Single cells are easy to obtain. They can be coughed from the lungs or be found in urine samples, the fluid around the spine or fluid that may accumulate in the chest or abdominal cavities. Cells can be scraped from the skin's surface or from other organs such as from the cervix for a Pap smear test.

We perform a number of blood tests in patients with cancer. Except in the case of cancers of blood cells, the leukaemias, we are usually not able to see circulating cancer cells in the blood since there are too few of them. The routine blood tests are to look for more indirect evidence of the effects of a tumour. In the future, we may be able to routinely detect the very small numbers of circulating solid tumour cells.

LOOKING AT CANCERS UNDER THE MICROSCOPE

What do we do with the piece of tissue once we have obtained it? Traditionally, we send it to a pathologist so that it can be looked at under a microscope and identified. (Taking a biopsy in order to diagnose the problem before surgery dates as far back as about 1900 in Germany.) The pathologist should be provided with as much information as possible to help put the tissue specimen into the context of the illness seen in the patient. The likelihood of a cancer occurring may differ depending on the patient's age or the site of a lump.

The pathologist classifies the cancer using internationally accepted groupings, depending on what is seen under the light microscope. The adoption of international conventions for naming tumours allows easier comparisons between pathologists and between the countries that record the incidence and out-comes of different tumour types. There can be differences of opinion between pathologists about which type a tumour seen under a microscope fits into. Those of us who treat tumours ask for a second opinion from our own pathologist if the original tumour was diagnosed elsewhere.

These differences of opinion surprise some patients who believe that, after a biopsy, their doctor should be able to tell them, beyond all reasonable doubt, whether they have cancer and what that cancer is. This is most often the case, but there may be a problem. It is not just the differing skill level of pathologists that allows a margin for error—although, as in any field, the more experienced pathologists are likely to be more accurate in diagnosis than those who have seen fewer cancers—there are other problems when identifying a cancer by looking at it under a microscope.

It can be difficult under the microscope to tell whether a lump is benign or malignant. You may not know from a single biopsy about local invasion or distant spread and it can be difficult to tell just by looking at cells whether they have crossed the line between normality and cancer.

Even if the lump is cancerous, is the small piece of a cancer that is being looked at representative of the rest of the tumour, which may vary from one section to another? In fact, sometimes, when a small biopsy specimen is looked at under the microscope it contains no cancerous tissue, even though the operator was certain that it came from the abnormal area that was being investigated. This can occur if a cancer is surrounded by inflammation and the biopsy from one corner, by bad luck, has hit only the surrounding inflamed tissue.

It is often easier to diagnose a cancer if the biopsy is taken from the primary site (i.e. its site of origin) rather than from a secondary site to which it has spread. This is because the cancer cells may look more like the organ from which they came. If a cancer cell is mature it may look very much like the cells of its organ of origin and then the diagnosis of the type of cancer is straightforward. If a cancer cell is primitive, or has not developed the distinctive specialised look of its parent cell type, it can be impossible to tell exactly where it has come from. The pathology report will say that it is a cancer, because of the appearance of the dividing cells, but may suggest a range of possible sites of origin.

More difficult still can be deciding how aggressive the tumour is by its appearance. There are rules for deciding the grade of a tumour which depend on such features as how many cells in a specimen are dividing, or how much they look like the normal cells of the organ of origin. There will, however, always be specimens where there are cells on the borderline between two grades and here interpretations may differ.

Sometimes pathologists have divided tumours into subtypes to reflect their expected clinical behaviour. Cancers of lymph glands provide a good example. The grade of a tumour depends on such features as the size of the cells and the pattern of the cells, whether they form sheets of cells or clumps. It may be necessary to examine a whole gland rather than just a small piece to detect the pattern of the cells, and it can be difficult to tell which pattern predominates. Sometimes new patterns are identified as distinctive subgroups with different outcomes and pathologists must learn to identify these.

While we are talking about lymph glands, it can be important to know whether some tumours have developed secondary spread to the lymph glands draining the area where the tumour originated. The likelihood of breast cancer returning can be judged on whether the lymph glands beneath the arm are involved at the time of the breast surgery. If a whole gland is replaced by cancer, deciding about spread of the tumour is easy and reproducible between pathologists. If, however, there is just a tiny clump of cells in a gland, detection by looking at it under a microscope may depend on how many slices of the gland the pathologist looks at. The pathologist can't look at every cell in every surgical specimen that is sent.

Which parts of the specimen are examined may also be important in determining whether the surgeon has completely removed the tumour or whether cancer cells are seen at the edges of the surgical specimen, indicating that more extensive surgery may be necessary. In the skin cancer, melanoma, this is important information as you must remove it all to have a chance for cure. In melanomas, the thickness of the cancer must also be reported since this is a determinant of whether it will come back.

The pathologist looks at the tissue sections after they have been stained by dyes. The dyes highlight different cells and parts of the cell as different colours to aid identification. There are routine rapid stains, and then there are special stains which look for particular targets—these help to identify specific tumours which are known to contain those chemical targets. Other methods to assist the pathologist, in addition to looking at the structure of a tumour under a microscope, include immunohistochemistry, DNA content analysis and molecular genetics.

Immunohistochemistry

This term has not come from a 'Scrabble' dictionary but is a word made from several others. The 'immuno' part of the word is the key since the colouring of cells makes use of proteins that are part of the immune system. Each cell has on its surface proteins called antigens which can be recognised by antibodies. Antibodies usually form part of the body's immune system by recognising antigens that are foreign to the body. The fact that antibodies attach to antigens can be used by the pathologist who puts the antibody on a slide to bind to the cells which display the antigen that it targets. The antibody to a particular cell can be given a fluorescent tag or can be coloured so that those cells will stand out when looked at under a microscope. If there are single cells, the number of cells with fluorescent tags can be counted as they flow along a tube in a machine called a flow cytometer.

Another use for such a technique is to distinguish benign from cancerous cells if there are certain antigens associated only with cancerous cells. With cancers of lymph glands, the cells will all contain the same type of antigens, whereas normal lymph node cells have a mixture of antigens.

The major use of immunohistochemistry has not been to make the first diagnosis of a cancer but to classify a cancer into subgroups. Again we can use the example of lymphomas where each subtype will have a different pattern of antigens on its cell surface. We return to lymphomas in Chapter 7.

Another important use of this technique is in trying to identify the primary site of origin of cells biopsied from distant secondary sites where it is difficult to determine the site of the primary. They should display antigens on their surface which are characteristic of their tissue of origin, irrespective of where that is.

DNA content analysis

We have talked about cancer being due to disruptions in genes and chromosomes. It is not surprising, therefore, that imaging the DNA content of cells could be useful in characterising cancer. First, cancer cells can have changes in chromosome numbers. This type of change is more often seen with more aggressive cancers. Second, more cancer cells will be dividing than in normal tissue. Just before a cell divides it must duplicate its DNA. In both cases the DNA can be stained and the affected cells seen either by a microscope or flow cytometer.

Analysing genes

At an even finer level than staining DNA, the sequence of the bases, the alphabet, that makes up the genes, can be read by techniques that continue to be developed. The results are far more definite and require less interpretation. They are also more sensitive, which means that a very little disease can be detected compared with the amount needed to be seen by the light microscope.

A detailed discussion of the various techniques is not necessary for an understanding of how cancer is diagnosed, but a brief description provides insight into the clever ways in which researchers have solved problems in this area. Let us take the example of wanting to detect changes in the sequences of DNA, either deletions of lengths of it or rearrangements of the bases. DNA is extracted from the cells and cut up into lengths by enzymes (proteins that digest tissues at various points). These DNA single strands are then sorted into lengths by passing an electric current through a gel. The current makes some sections of DNA travel further than others, depending on their size. The various strips of DNA are then 'blotted' onto a membrane and, to detect a particular sequence of interest, probes are prepared. For DNA these probes are simply single strands of DNA of known sequence that are labelled so that they can be detected if they find and join with a complementary single strand of the cell's DNA on the membrane.

This technique is called Southern blot hybridisation after the man who developed it. Similar techniques for RNA and proteins have been designated Northern and Western blots respectively. These techniques really have given new direction to the analysis of tumours and the genetic changes underlying them.

The use of single-stranded probes to detect DNA or RNA by binding or hybridising with complementary strands in the cells being analysed can also be applied to tissue sections. This is known as *in situ* hybridisation. It applies probes to tissue sections so that the distribution of the cells with the sequences of interest that may mark them as cancerous can be seen within a slice of tissue. It is often used to detect the presence of DNA or RNA from viruses that may be found in some types of cancerous cells.

A further variation of this technique, known as FISH (fluorescent *in situ* hybridisation), involves preparing DNA probes to detect chromosome abnormalities in pieces of chromosome visible under the light microscope. These can be tagged with a fluorescent chemical which enables the abnormality to be seen under a microscope in cells that are about to divide. The chromosomes are most easily visible when they arrange themselves just before the cell divides.

A final piece of cleverness which has made an enormous impact on research solves the problem of having only a tiny amount of the DNA or RNA that you want to detect—either because there are only a few copies of a sequence in a large number of cells or only a tiny amount of tissue. The obvious solution is to amplify the sequence required by making multiple copies of it. To do this for DNA, for example, small pieces of manufactured DNA are attached to either end of the sequence to be copied. This attached DNA initiates the replication of the whole DNA strand when you add DNA polymerase which assists the incorporation of bases in order to make copies of the DNA sequence of interest. The technique is termed PCR or the polymerase chain reaction.

Making multiple copies of the DNA or RNA sequence of interest allows easier detection of the presence of that sequence. This may be important for diagnosis. It also enables detailed study of the composition of the strand. Even if there is only a small amount of DNA present in old degraded pathology specimens this technique can produce more to allow further study. Fans of the movie 'Jurassic Park' will see the potential of this technique for amplifying small amounts of prehistoric DNA from archaeological specimens.

Although they are complex, I have discussed these techniques because they are allowing molecular biologists to study cancer right down to the level of the DNA molecules. We have seen how this can be applied to the diagnosis of cancer; it also provides the possibility of influencing the processes at this level as a treatment of the disease.

Electron microscopy

Light provides a magnification which allows the pathologist to identify most tumours. In a few cases the electron microscope can be useful because it gives the pathologist further magnification of small structures within a cell. But an electron microscope is expensive and slow and requires skilled operators. Also, not many tumours have structures that can be seen only by electron microscopy and are unique enough to make a diagnosis. Sometimes, though, it may be useful to see virus particles in association with a tumour and some tumours are characterised by small granules which can be seen under this extreme magnification.

IS THERE A BLOOD TEST FOR CANCER?

We have already discovered that cancer cells can travel from their primary site to secondary sites through the bloodstream. We often perform blood tests on patients as part of their diagnosis of cancer and to monitor their treatment. This leads some patients to assume that we can see the cancer cells in the blood. I have already dispelled that notion. There are so few cancer cells at any one time that we cannot detect them simply by examining the blood under a microscope.

Some of the tests discussed above could be used to detect minimal disease by amplifying the DNA that is present. Much research is being done to enable detection of cancers by simple blood tests using a variety of techniques designed to detect the unique characteristics of tumours.

In a few situations, the tumour produces chemicals that can be measured in the blood. These substances act as markers of disease activity. Often, they allow detection of the tumour before there are enough cells for it to be felt or seen by scans. These markers in the blood can be used to help make the diagnosis, follow the progress of treatment and detect a relapse of the cancer. Unfortunately, it is only in rare cases that cancers are associated with markers that are specific to them. The first example was the description in 1848 by Bence Jones of proteins associated with myeloma (a cancer of the plasma cells in the bone marrow that produce proteins). They are still called Bence Jones proteins. Decades later, examples include the markers β HCG and α fetoprotein in testicular cancer, and PSA or prostate specific antigen in prostate cancer. We return to these and others when discussing specific tumours and screening.

THE IMAGING OF CANCER

Pathology tests are most important for making a definitive diagnosis of cancer, but being able to see a cancer when you can't feel it is also vital. Techniques that image cancers can help in diagnosis and in gauging the extent of spread of a tumour. Serial x-rays or scans are useful in following the progress of a tumour. There are many different types of scans, all giving different perspectives on a cancer.

In moving from pathology tests to imaging tests you may have thought 'and now for something completely different', but now that imaging can detect chemical changes within a cell the distinction between the two approaches is becoming blurred.

Life is but a walking shadow . . .

This famous line from the tragedy of *Macbeth* by William Shakespeare could also describe life from the perspective of a radiologist. Most imaging techniques are just shadows on photographic paper that require interpretation. X-rays and scans are not the ultimate arbiters of the presence of cancer. They do not see all. It is sobering to realise that many scans are only able to detect cancers when they reach 1 centimetre in size, although CT scans of the lung may detect small deposits of 3–4 millimetres. Even then, as we found in Chapter 1, we are dealing with something like a billion cells. Also, as I explain to my patients, if the tumour is in sheets rather than lumps, a scan may look right through it.

There are many different types of scans. Cancers can be seen on plain x-rays, CT scans, MRI scans, ultrasounds, nuclear medicine scans and PET scans among others. Which scan do we choose? The answer changes constantly as improved scanning techniques are developed. The choice will depend on which organ we wish to scan, the availability of the scan, expertise to interpret it and the budget to afford it. The accuracy of a scanning technique depends on its sensitivity, the percentage of cancers that are detected when they are present, and its specificity (the percentage of patients without cancer who are identified as such).

Over the years we have seen one type of scan replace another. For example, the gold standard test for detecting a cancer pressing on the spinal cord used to be a myelogram. This involved injecting contrast material into the fluid which surrounds the spinal cord and taking x-rays as the patient was tilted so that the contrast ran up beside the spinal cord. This invasive procedure has now been replaced by the MRI scan which, in a non-invasive procedure, can image the whole cord and give accurate information about the size of the lump. For looking at abdominal lymph glands, CT scans have largely replaced lymphograms which required contrast to be injected into the small lymphatic channels in the webbing of the feet, a dying art. A nuclear medicine bone scan can detect hot spots in bones but can't tell what causes them. Hot spots on a bone scan could be at sites of fractures, cancers or inflammation. To look further at the area, plain x-rays can be used. Better, however, is a CT scan and better still an MRI scan.

Finding out where a cancer is and how extensive it is—what we call staging a cancer—is important for two reasons. First, it will help determine the best treatment. A cancer that is of limited size and has not spread may be curable by surgery, whereas operating would not help more extensive disease. Second, the extent of a tumour is helpful in predicting its outcome, or prognosis. Let us look at each type of imaging technique so that you can understand their uses and limitations in the diagnosis and management of cancers.

Plain x-ray films

Wilhelm Roentgen, a German physicist, discovered x-rays in 1895 and was subsequently awarded the Nobel Prize. For medical imaging, an x-ray beam is passed through the body and produces an image on a film. A well known example is the plain chest x-ray where the dense bones appear white, while the air-containing lung looks black (Figure 3.1). The 'shadow' of the heart is also seen in the centre of the film and its size can be measured. A good overall picture is seen but for greater detail other techniques are used. Although it is easy to see the difference between dense bone and lung, it may not be easy to distinguish more subtle differences between soft tissues or to see through tissues that lie one behind the other.

A similar technique is employed to image the breasts. Mammography is the only radiographic technique routinely used to screen for cancers (Figure 3.2). Good images are obtained with low radiation doses. Mammography is not invasive and is relatively inexpensive—necessary if a test is to be used for screening people who are well but at risk.

A variation on the plain x-ray is the tomograph (from the Greek for section). Here, if the x-ray tube is swung around a fixed slice, everything will be blurred except that slice and a picture of a 'cut' through the tissue will result. A particular section of the body where there is a point of interest can be imaged.

Many organs that cannot be seen by routine x-ray proce-

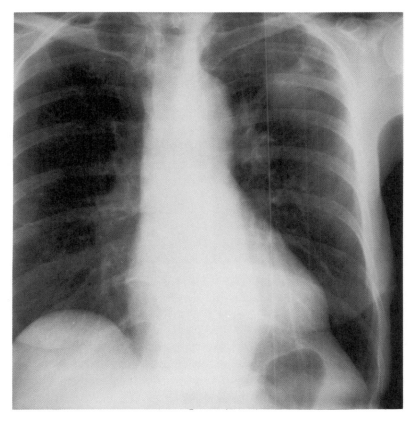

Figure 3.1 Chest x-ray showing the heart shadow in the centre and a cancer near the top of the left lung (right side of photograph)

dures can be made visible by the use of substances which are opaque to x-rays and which provide contrast between the tissues and the dense substances. The best known examples are for imaging the bowels; barium or gastrograffin can be swallowed or given by enema to outline the wall of the bowel and look for irregularities. Contrast media can also be injected into joints for arthrograms, into the fluid surrounding the spine for myelograms looking at the spinal cord, or into blood vessels for angiograms to look for blockages in vessels or perhaps to image

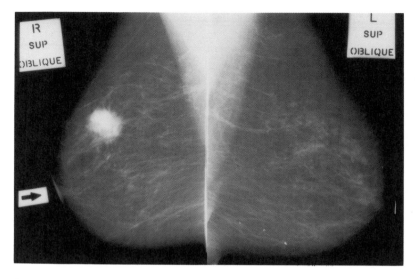

Figure 3.2 Mammogram showing views of the left and right breasts for comparison and a typical star-shaped cancer in the right breast

the vessels supplying cancers. As the contrast is injected, moving images can be viewed and recorded on film or videotape or seen on fluoroscopes. Sample views can be captured on film as a record of any abnormality seen.

CT scans

Popularly known as a CAT scan, this method of imaging has nothing to do with feline pets but is an acronym for computerised axial tomography. A computer analyses the data from thin x-ray beams passed through cross-sections of the body as the patient lies on a table and is passed through a doughnut-shaped machine. The computer can reconstruct the image in any plane, so it is more properly known now as a CT scan. It allows slices to be examined with great definition between soft tissues. Contrast substances can also be given to allow identification of hollow organs like the bowel, or vascular organs if intravenous contrast is given. With the new helical CT scanners,

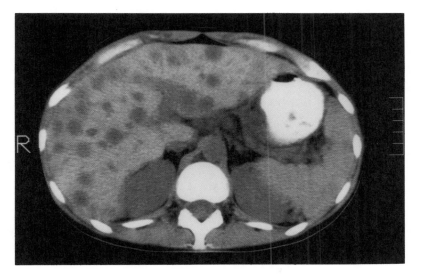

Figure 3.3 CT scan cross-section of the abdomen showing the liver
with multiple deposits of cancer

information about various sections of the body can be collected
more quickly than was possible with the older slice-by-slice
method.

CT scanning allows us to look inside the body at any level.
When the lungs are imaged, the blood vessels can be seen and
any abnormality such as a cancer can be examined in its three
dimensions. It is possible to see smaller cancers than on a plain
x-ray. You can see and separate out the structures that lie in
front of or behind the heart. This may be very useful for
determining whether a lung cancer, for example, has spread to
the lymph glands in the centre of the chest, making the cancer
inoperable. CT scans allowed us to see the organs in the
abdomen, which were difficult to visualise in any other way.
The CT scan is excellent at looking at the liver, pancreas,
kidneys and adrenal glands as well as lymph glands at the back
of the abdomen (Figure 3.3).

As mentioned above, sheets of tumour rather than lumps
may be missed, but their presence may be suggested if they

make the bowel loops appear rigid or if they are associated with fluid production. The scan can be set to make it easier to see the soft tissues or, if necessary, the bones. Surgical clips or metal will cause shadows which obscure the detail of the surrounding soft tissues.

CT scans are also very good at looking at the brain where cancers could otherwise only be imaged on plain x-rays if they contained calcium, or indirectly if the blood vessels supplying them could be injected with contrast. The major problem with CT scans of the head is at the edges of the brain which can be overshadowed by being close to the dense bone of the skull.

CT scans, being non-invasive, have superseded many of the lymphograms and angiograms and have even reduced the need for surgical exploration. Once all the data has been stored in the computer it can be reconstructed into three-dimensional images. This is proving particularly useful in planning radiotherapy fields that will adequately encompass tumours while sparing normal tissues (see Chapter 5). Virtual reality reconstructions of organs are also possible with this technology.

MRI scans

Magnetic resonance imaging was developed after CT scans and does not use x-rays. The technique hinges on the fact that the atomic nuclei of various elements, like the hydrogen in water, have magnetic properties. This alone may enable differentiation between tissues of different water content. If the nuclei are placed in a magnetic field they all line up like compass needles in the same direction. This effect of the magnetic field can be measured. If you expose different parts of the body to different magnetic fields they will produce different signals, allowing you to tell where the part is in relation to another part. A radiofrequency pulse disturbs the field, and the time it takes for return of the atom's magnetisation to normal varies depending on the type of tissue, creating another way of distinguishing between tissues. A computer can take this information and reconstruct images of slices of the body in any direction, just like a CT scan.

A contrast agent called gadolinium can be injected into a patient's veins and used with MRI to highlight the difference between a cancer and the swelling in the surrounding tissue, which can be difficult to distinguish with other imaging techniques. It can also show breaches in the barrier between the brain and blood, useful in detecting tumours of the brain or its lining.

MRI scans have an advantage over CT scans in the brain where the border between the brain and the skull is seen more clearly. The spinal cord can be imaged without having to inject contrast into the spinal fluid, and it is easy to see an image of the length of the spinal cord (Figure 3.4).

MRI scans have proved to be particularly useful in the head, neck and pelvis because of high contrast between soft tissues and the difference in signal intensity between fibrosis and recurrent tumour. The use of MRI in the breast is being explored.

MRS (magnetic resonance spectroscopy) is a related technique based on the fact that nuclei associated with different chemicals emit different signals. MRS can be used to study differences in tissues based on differences in their chemistry at the level of the cell, much like PET scanning (discussed below).

Ultrasound

The principles of ultrasound are similar to those used for depth sounding to find submarines or sunken treasure in the sea. In fact, the clinical ultrasound was developed from equipment that used high-frequency sound waves to test the continuity of welded joints. Essentially, sound travels through tissue and is reflected back when it reaches an interface between two tissues. Some tissues, such as gas and bone, are impenetrable and so limit the use of the technique. Also, the interpretation of what is seen is very dependent on the operator. On the other hand, an ultrasound can be done instantly and cheaply, and doesn't require injections of contrast or exposure of patients to x-rays (Figure 3.5).

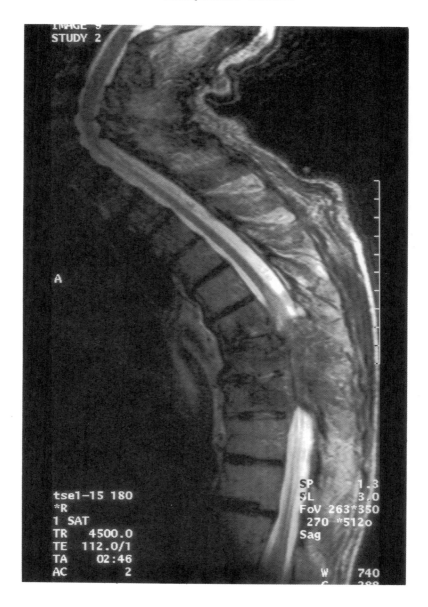

Figure 3.4 MRI scan of the spine and spinal cord showing a large cancer pressing on the spinal cord

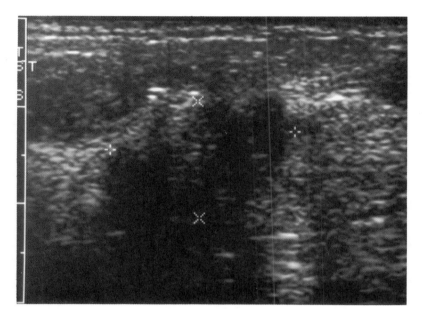

Figure 3.5 Ultrasound of the breast showing the shadow from a cancer, marked by the crosses

Ultrasound is good for looking at dilated bile ducts and what is obstructing them. In the liver, cysts containing fluid can be distinguished from solid lumps. Masses in the breast can also be measured and solid lumps can be separated from cysts containing fluid. Kidney, pancreatic and ovarian masses can be easily explored. It is a good technique for guiding needles for biopsies since it can be done in real time without radiation.

A variation on the ultrasound is colour Doppler sonography, where a colour can be assigned on the image to the blood flow, depending on its direction and speed, without the use of contrast. This can detect obstructions to blood flow and can also see the abnormal blood vessels that are found in some cancers.

Nuclear medicine imaging

Nuclear medicine techniques make use of the differences in function between different tissues, or sites in a tissue.

Figure 3.6
Whole body bone scan—the dark spots in the bones are deposits of cancer

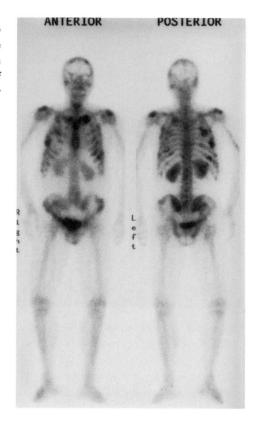

Radioactive tracers can be taken up by tissues and their presence detected by a camera that picks up the gamma rays they give off. The dose of radiation to the patient is minute and the tracer decays quickly to become harmless.

Let me illustrate this with the nuclear bone scan. Bones take up phosphate which can be labelled with radioactive tracer called technetium. A technetium labelled phosphate is taken up where new bone is being produced. This may be at the site of a tumour or a fracture or inflammation and will show as a hot spot in the bone when a picture is taken by the gamma camera (Figure 3.6).

The scan can't give the cause of the hot spot. That will have to be determined by what is most likely from taking a history and examining the patient. However, in the case of a cancer, it is more sensitive than a plain x-ray for detecting its presence. The area indicated as hot could then be imaged by MRI or CT to determine its nature more precisely.

Like a plain x-ray, the bone scan gives just a two-dimensional image. However, a tomographic technique called SPECT (single photon emission computed tomography) can give cross-sectional pictures using a similar technique to that described for the plain x-ray tomograms.

Other isotopes can be used to image other organs such as the breast, liver or lymph nodes. In future, labelling antigens on the surface of cancer cells with a radioactive tracer will allow very small cancers to be detected.

PET scans

PET scans, again nothing to do with pets, are positron emission tomographs. They differentiate tissues by the different chemical changes occurring in their cells. For example, tissues can be differentiated by how they break down sugar. PET is a scan that relies on the function of a tissue rather than its relation in space to another tissue. In cancers, for example, glucose break-down is followed by using FDG, where a radioactive fluoride tagged glucose which emits gamma rays enters the cells and takes part in the chemical glucose utilisation process. A computer can use the information from gamma cameras to construct an image. The beauty of this type of image is that the degree of glucose utilisation correlates with the aggressiveness of the tumour. It is also possible to follow the chemical changes caused to the tumour by drug therapy. Chemical changes will often occur well before structural changes in tissue.

PET is very expensive and the daily production of the radioactive tracers requires access to a cyclotron or generator which may limit use of this type of scan.

Other uses of radiological techniques

The techniques used by radiologists are not only useful for imaging. We have mentioned the use of ultrasounds to guide biopsy needles. CT scans can also be used for this. Fluid can be drained from body cavities, using ultrasound or CT to guide the needle.

Radiologists are used to putting catheters into arteries to inject contrast. The same technique can be adapted to block the blood supply to a cancer or insert a tube into the artery feeding the liver to inject drugs. When cancers cause blocking of bile ducts or kidneys these can be drained through the skin by tubes guided into position by radiological imaging.

THE WILL ROGERS PHENOMENON

I end this chapter with a cautionary tale told by Feinstein and colleagues in the *New England Journal of Medicine*. It illustrates why we can't assume that improvements in survival from cancer from one decade to the next are necessarily due to improved treatments.

Will Rogers was an American comedian who quipped that 'when the Oakies moved to California it increased the IQ of both states'. How does this insult to the Californians relate to cancer? Imagine that you have a tumour that is at a higher stage if there are lung secondaries and at a lower stage if there are not. You also have data showing that the outcomes for both stages have improved over the decades. Can you assume that the treatments have become better? No. For example, the treatment may not have improved but what did happen was that the CT scan was introduced. What this did was to move the worst of the lower-stage patients—who really had lung secondaries but they were too small to see on x-ray and could only be seen on CT scan—up into the higher-stage group. This would improve the apparent outcome of the lower stages since the worst of the patients had been removed. However, it would also improve the outcome of the higher-stage group which now contained patients with only minimal lung metastases.

Keep this story about the impact of the improved detection of cancer in mind when we talk about clinical trials of treatments in Chapter 9. Meanwhile, if detecting cancer early improves the outcome, what strategies can we use to do this?

SUMMARY

The definitive test for cancer is to take some tissue for a biopsy. Newer techniques have meant that smaller and smaller tissue samples are needed. Special stains can be used to distinguish a cancer cell from a normal cell. More sensitive tests are being developed that characterise a cell by analysing its DNA, RNA or proteins. Cancers can be viewed in three dimensions as plain x-rays give way to CT and MRI scans and nuclear medicine techniques.

4

Getting it early

A stitch in time saves nine.

—*Proverb*

Screening for cancer means trying to detect the cancer when it is small, before it has caused symptoms. Experience shows that we get better results with tumours that have not spread. The hope is that screening people at risk of cancer will improve the chances that treatment will work and that more people will be cured. This sounds like a good idea and it can be, but so far it has been of benefit for only a few cancers.

The concept of screening also applies at an earlier life stage to detect people at risk by looking for genes and gene mutations that increase their likelihood of developing cancer. I discuss this at the end of this chapter.

For screening of a population to be useful, there must be a test that will detect the cancer early in a large proportion of cases and a treatment that is more effective if commenced earlier. Moreover, the test has to be cheap and easy, since it has to be applied to a large population of people, most of whom will be well. Also, a screening test must have a high chance of detecting disease if it is present and a low chance of giving a positive result if the disease is not there.

Before we look at specific cancers I want to discuss the likely benefits and disadvantages of screening so that you will be able to decide whether it is worthwhile, rather than just accepting that if a test becomes available it should be used. Screening a whole population is expensive and the cost must be justified by the benefit to the community. Screening won't be helpful, for example, if a slowly growing localised cancer would still be curable even if it was left until it became obvious. Conversely, a cancer that has already spread before the primary cancer can be detected will not benefit from a screening program either.

TESTING WHETHER SCREENING WORKS

How would you go about evaluating a screening program? First, you obviously hope that a reasonable percentage of the population accept the offer to be screened. You could then look at the yield of cancers from the population that was screened, since in the first round of screening you would expect it to be higher than that for the rest of the population. If the screening is effective, you should be detecting extra cases that otherwise would not be found until later when they were more advanced. This also means there should be a higher occurrence of early-stage disease in the screened group.

The endpoint that you really want to influence by screening is survival. You would like to show that the survival of the group who were screened is better than that of the unscreened population. Comparing a screened and unscreened group, however, is not that simple. Although it seems straightforward there are biases that can inappropriately affect the result.

For example, there is what is called a lead time bias. Survival is measured from the time of diagnosis. Because screening makes the diagnosis earlier, the survival of the screened group is automatically extended by that earlier time, irrespective of the date of death. Furthermore, the screen-detected group should contain more slow-growing cancers than the rest of the population because slower-growing cancers will spend a longer time before they cause symptoms than faster-growing cancers, and therefore have more chance of being detected by a screening program. The slower-growing cancers should do better than the faster-growing ones.

One other factor is that screening may detect some early cases that would never have progressed to causing symptoms in the lifetime of the patient. Also, the individuals who accept screening are likely to be more concerned about their health than the population at large, another difference which could influence the outcome of this group.

We can allow for some of these situations. We usually make a valid comparison by comparing the rates of cancer deaths in each group. This is taken from the start of the screening program and won't be subject to any of the biases discussed above. We revisit some of these problems when deciding which cancers warrant population screening programs.

The best way to assess a screening program is to set up a trial where a group of people is allocated, by chance, either to screening or not, and both groups followed for long enough to see if there is a difference in cancer deaths. There are other methods of comparison, such as screening a group and then trying to obtain a matched group that isn't being screened, but the method of randomly allocating patients in advance is most likely to result in groups that are truly comparable in all respects except that one group has been screened.

One other decision that will alter the outcome of screening is how often screening should be done. This will differ from one cancer to the next, depending on how quickly a cancer progresses from detectable without symptoms to detectable because of symptoms. Also, if screening is to be beneficial, there must be a sound system for following up the positive cases to initiate treatment as required.

POSSIBLE DISADVANTAGES OF SCREENING

The potential advantage of screening is to save lives by detecting a cancer earlier and being able to cure it. The treatment may also be cheaper and less burdensome for early-stage disease. The potential disadvantages begin with the screening test itself. For example, the exposure to radiation from multiple x-rays could increase the risk of second cancers. In another example, although rare, there is a small risk of puncturing the bowel during a colonoscopy to detect early bowel cancer. Screening tests have been refined to minimise the risk. The cumulative dose from having repeated mammograms is low. However, no screening test would be justified if the risks outweighed the potential benefit.

Nothing in this world is 100 per cent perfect and screening tests can yield results that are falsely positive. This may, occasionally, expose a patient to unnecessary physical procedures, such as a biopsy. More, though, it could increase anxiety or depression over having cancer detected. It is even suggested that spreading information about screening may do the same, although little research has been done on this. Again, if the chance of a false positive is small, it won't affect the decision to screen, but is one of the factors to be balanced with the benefits. Obviously, false negatives can be inappropriately re-assuring, but people should understand that a negative test gives no guarantees about the future and should not result in ignoring symptoms or failing to have the test repeated in the future.

Screening detects cases that would not be known without it. This may mean that some cases are detected that would never have progressed in the patient's lifetime. This is particularly a problem if the screening test is detecting changes that precede cancer, rather than early cancer, but we may also know little about the natural history of very slow-growing cancers. I return to this point when discussing screening for prostate cancer later in this chapter.

Some of you may feel uncomfortable about evaluating a health program on the basis of cost to the community. However, it is important because there will never be enough money to do everything and we must ensure that we are using the available money in the most cost-effective way. We would not want to put all our resources into screening for a whole range of cancers if that meant there was no money for prevention programs or curative treatments. One way of making population screening more cost-effective is to target the groups of people at highest risk, rather than screen everyone. This also limits those who will benefit, however. Note that the effectiveness of screening is being judged here on a population basis, not predicting whether a particular individual will benefit. I illustrate many of these points in the discussion that follows.

BREAST CANCER SCREENING

The best studied screening program is that for breast cancer. But, despite monitoring more than half a million women on randomised trials and many more on non-randomised screening programs, some of the details of how best to screen remain unclear. There are eight large randomised trials. The first began in 1963, although the technique of mammography was described 50 years earlier. The earliest trials can now compare deaths in the screened and unscreened groups over ten years.

The trials differ from each other in important ways. First, the age at which women are screened varies. Most trials cover women in their fifties and sixties, while only some include women in their forties. The number of women in their seventies is relatively small. What is involved in screening also differs between studies. Some studies use only one-view mammography while others use two-view techniques. The latest of the large studies was designed to evaluate the addition of mammography to clinical breast examination. Finally, the interval between screening examinations has varied from twelve months to 33 months. I have given these details because this enormous amount of data is open to varying interpretations and it is important to understand the reason for this.

Steering a middle course, I would suggest there is no doubt that screening for breast cancer is associated with a definite decrease in deaths in women in their fifties and sixties, and they should be encouraged to participate in screening programs. Harris and colleagues have estimated that between two and seven women would have their lives saved by screening for every 10 000 women between 50 and 60 years who were screened. Although numbers are smaller in the over-seventies group, women who are still fit are being screened.

Fewer women between 40 and 50 years are being screened and most of the trials have not been set up specifically to assess the benefits of screening in this age group. In younger women, screening is technically more difficult because the breasts are denser and it is more difficult to see a thickening that may suggest an early cancer. Overall, any improvement in mortality in the 40 to 50 years age group has been borderline and routine screening of this group has not been recommended.

The trials have also suggested that adding a clinical breast examination to the mammography results in an additional reduction in mortality. The frequency of screening should probably be at least every two years. If screening takes place every two years, it would make sense to have a doctor carry out a good clinical examination of the breast annually.

I have not mentioned breast self-examination to date. Although women should be encouraged to take an active interest in their health and present early with a lump, it has been difficult to show that breast self-examination results in the earlier detection that reduces mortality in a population. However, it can certainly benefit individual women in identifying their breast cancer.

These recommendations are for the population at large. There are high-risk groups where more frequent and earlier screening would be prudent. Examples include women with a strong family history of breast cancer. Screening earlier than 50 would certainly be recommended for a woman whose mother had a breast cancer at a young age.

SCREENING FOR CANCER OF THE CERVIX

Cancer of the cervix is the second most common cancer in the world and is often the leading cause of cancer death in women in economically poor countries. Its incidence is higher in sexually promiscuous women and it is strongly related to human papilloma virus infection. To understand why screening is possible for cervical cancer you need to know that changes in the cells lining the outer cervix can occur years before invasive cancer develops. These changes are designated CIN 1,2 and 3: CIN stands for cervical intraepithelial neoplasia and the numbers indicate the extent of the abnormality. There is more than fifteen years' difference between the average age at which women are found to have CIN and the average age of invasive cancer, which shows how slow the progression is. Also, not all women with CIN will progress and in some the changes have become better.

The screening test is simple and inexpensive. A speculum is inserted into the vagina so the cervix can be seen. A cotton swab is used to take a sample from the inside of the cervix and a wooden or plastic spatula is used to scrape the outside of the cervix and the sample smeared onto a glass slide. Abnormalities may be monitored simply by repeating the smear test, or followed by further visualisation and biopsy if more severe. Treatment may range from locally destroying the affected area to a hysterectomy for more advanced disease.

The Pap smear was introduced in the 1930s by George Papanicolaou. The use of the test was adopted so quickly that it was not possible to set up randomised clinical trials, as with breast cancer. We have had to rely on changes in mortality in regions over time after the introduction of the Pap test and on case-control studies where each participant in a population that has had screening is compared with a matched case in an unscreened population. This can give a biased comparison if the screened group is from a higher socioeconomic group of more motivated women who may have lower mortality anyway.

However, the reduction in mortality is impressive with estimations of up to 90 per cent reduction in deaths from the disease.

There is some uncertainty about the age of screening. Most groups recommend that screening begin at eighteen years or when a woman becomes sexually active. Because mortality increases with advancing age, it is difficult to suggest not screening older women. As for the screening frequency, most would recommend yearly tests until there are three negative tests, then every three years or at the physician's discretion.

Screening may lead to overdiagnosis if very early lesions are treated. Perhaps the lesions associated with specific types of papilloma virus are more likely to progress. However, the benefit has been shown to be such that the aim should be to screen all adult women for cancer of the cervix.

There are other cancers for which screening is advocated and this is being performed in some areas but the evidence of efficacy and cost benefit is more difficult to assess.

SCREENING FOR CANCER OF THE LARGE BOWEL

Large bowel cancer is a suitable cancer to consider for screening because it has a precancerous abnormality called an adenoma which often appears as a polyp or outgrowth of the lining of the bowel wall. There is usually a long time before cancer develops. Survival after an operation for bowel cancer does depend on the stage of the disease—that is, on how far through the bowel wall the cancer has penetrated—and so early detection, even after cancer has developed, can be important.

A variety of tests or combinations of tests could be used to screen for bowel cancer. The simplest and most inexpensive test, and therefore a promising candidate for screening a whole population, is the faecal occult blood test. This uses chemicals to test whether there are trace amounts of blood, which would not otherwise be seen, in the bowel motions. Patients are sent home with test kits and test three bowel actions for the presence of blood. If the test involves adding water to the sample, this increases the sensitivity of the test but also increases the possibility of a test being falsely positive.

Tests to visualise the bowel include a sigmoidoscopy where a doctor in an office setting can examine the lining of the lower bowel by introducing a tube with a light. This extends what can be palpated by examining the lower bowel with a finger but reaches only the lower portion of the large bowel. An air contrast barium enema, where a contrast material is introduced into the bowel and x-rays taken, can visualise the whole bowel. Likewise, a colonoscopy involves introducing a long flexible lighted tube to examine the whole bowel, but requires appropriate bowel preparation, and usually needs sedation in a day procedure area. It is the most risky of the procedures, with about a one-in-one-thousand chance of breaching the bowel wall, but also the most thorough. It is my experience that patients who have had both colonoscopies and barium studies usually prefer the former. The tests that look at the bowel are often advocated in combination with the faecal occult blood test for screening.

There are currently three large randomised controlled trials of screening using faecal occult blood tests. All show a reduction in bowel cancer death rates despite the relatively low sensitivity, or pick-up rate, when disease is present. One study has reported a 33 per cent reduction in mortality for patients having annual tests, although four in ten patients had had at least one colonoscopy. Many studies show that a screened group has earlier-stage cancers. A positive test will mean that a patient will go on to have a colonoscopy to find the cancer. This is where the expense comes in.

The use of sigmoidoscopies for screening has been supported by case-controlled studies that show a 60 per cent reduction in mortality. There are no controlled studies of screening with barium enemas or colonoscopies.

It is difficult to make recommendations from these results and which tests to use will ultimately be decided between patients and their doctor. It would seem reasonable that people

50 years old and over could be screened with a faecal occult blood test each year. The pick-up rate could be increased if a sigmoidoscopy was added every three to five years, but this adds complexity to a population screening program. Patients who have blood detected in the faeces would be further examined with a colonoscopy. Benign lesions such as haemorrhoids may be the cause of the bleeding and these can be easily treated. Follow-up colonoscopies may be required if polyps are found, or postoperatively to check the bowel after an early large bowel cancer has been removed.

Again, these are the facts that need to be considered if recommending that whole populations be screened. Individuals who are particularly at risk—because of a strong family history, for example—will in general be followed from an earlier age and more aggressively.

SCREENING FOR PROSTATE CANCER

Now we enter the grey zone. Before discussing screening for prostate cancer, I need to give you some details about the behaviour of this cancer. First, prostate cancer is not always a disease that causes death. Many prostate cancers are not aggressive and progress very slowly. It is estimated that three in ten men over 50 years will have very small clusters of prostate cancer cells that are doing them no harm. This increases with age to nearly two-thirds of men over 75 years. They have microscopic evidence of prostate cancer which may just sit there and never cause them a problem. On other occasions, when the cancer is more aggressive, it can spread early and the outcome is poor.

The problem is that screening will detect many cases of early disease where we simply don't know what the outcome will be. If all these men were subjected to treatment by surgical removal of the prostate or high doses of radiotherapy to the prostate, many patients would be treated unnecessarily. What is worse, two of the common side effects of these treatments are difficulty controlling the bladder and impotence. Even when prostate cancer is causing symptoms, if it is localised, watching it can achieve similar results in some patients to radical treatments, without the side effects. We don't have randomised trials to compare treatment policies, but one study estimated that radical treatment in a 65-year-old with slow-growing disease may improve survival by only one or two months, and by one year with aggressive disease. Patients will differ in what side effects they will tolerate in order to gain these benefits.

The screening tests that are available are a digital rectal examination (DRE, feeling the prostate by inserting a gloved finger into the lower bowel), an ultrasound done by the same route (TRUS or transrectal ultrasound) and a blood test for prostate specific antigen (PSA). Feeling the prostate is not particularly accurate as only about one-third of prostates that are positive on DRE will have cancer. TRUS only improves the situation a little, but is excellent for guiding biopsy needles. PSA can monitor the disease accurately and if elevated will fall to normal when the disease is treated, but it can be elevated in benign prostate enlargement and can be normal in one-third of men with localised prostate cancer.

A combination of PSA and DRE is commonly used with TRUS in selected cases, but no randomised trials are available. There is no evidence that survival and mortality are improved by population screening for prostate cancer. Given that it is unclear how to manage early prostate cancer, and yet its diagnosis could cause significant anxiety, there isn't a strong case at the moment for population screening for prostate cancer.

SCREENING FOR SKIN CANCER

The occurrence of skin cancer is increasing around the world. Melanoma, which is the most lethal form of skin cancer, is related to episodes of sunburn. If melanoma is detected early it can be cured by simple surgery. Screening begins with a public education campaign to increase awareness and seek attention for suspicious spots on the skin. No randomised studies have been done to determine the effectiveness of screening, but it may be difficult to find a control population who are not aware of a public education campaign.

In Australia (where melanoma incidence is high) there is some evidence that the incidence is increasing, but mortality is not increasing as quickly. One interpretation of this is that more people are seeking treatment for early lesions, which are being cured.

As with other tumour types, certain groups will require specific follow-up. There is an inherited condition, the dysplastic naevus syndrome, where individuals have more than their fair share of moles of many shapes and sizes, and a propensity to develop melanoma. This condition requires annual photography of the skin surface and the removal of any suspicious moles.

SCREENING FOR OTHER CANCERS

Screening of the population cannot at present be recommended for other cancers for a variety of reasons. Three prospective randomised trials and two case-controlled studies have shown no reduction in mortality with screening for lung cancer by routine x-ray or examination of the sputum for cancer cells.

Self-examination for cancer of the testicle has been advocated, but there is no precancerous abnormality to detect and the current very effective treatment means that even those who present with symptoms have a low death rate. This should not, however, deter individuals from seeking help early if they have symptoms.

Screening for stomach cancer has been used in Japan where there is a lot more of this cancer than in Western countries. There may be some benefit, but it is difficult to evaluate. Screening for stomach cancer requires barium studies which can be costly and expose the patient to radiation. Tests for ovarian cancer (ultrasound of the pelvis and a blood test, the CA–125) are not specific enough to suggest they will be useful. High-risk groups have been screened for bladder cancer by examining the urine for abnormal cells, but no reduction in mortality of screened over unscreened groups has been found.

GENETIC SCREENING

Genetic screening can assess the risk of individuals developing cancer during their lifetime. This type of screening differs markedly from that discussed above. The information will affect mortality if the cancer can be prevented from developing, or if it is one of the cancers where screening and early detection reduce mortality and intensive screening is implemented because of the increased risk. Genetic screening presents many dilemmas. The following illustration uses the example of breast cancer, but the implications will increasingly apply to other tumour types.

Family history is a recognised risk factor for breast cancer. We discussed earlier how a mutation in a tumour suppressor gene, although uncommon and associated with only 5–10 per cent of breast cancer cases, is associated with a very high risk of developing breast cancer during the woman's lifetime. A mutation in BRCA 1, for example, is associated with an 85 per cent lifetime risk of developing breast cancer. Most women with a family history will not have such a mutation and their lifetime risk of developing the disease does not exceed 30 per cent. The likelihood of breast cancer being genetically transmitted is increased in women with a history of multiple relatives with breast cancer, particularly if they get it at a young age.

Genetic testing may have profound implications for the individual tested, but also for other members of the family. Such testing should not occur without appropriate counselling. A woman may not wish to know what her lifetime risk of breast cancer is. Let us say we test a woman with a strong family history of breast cancer for BRCA 1. A negative test for a BRCA 1 mutation could mean that the woman has not inherited the family risk of breast cancer. This would be the case if we knew that a family member with breast cancer had a BRCA 1 mutation. Otherwise, a negative test could simply mean that a different gene mutation is responsible for that family's cancer. A negative test should not reassure the woman to such an extent that she does not participate in screening because she still has the risk of developing breast cancer, but not the very high risk associated with BRCA 1 mutations. We are assuming here that we have confidence in the accuracy of the tests.

If the cancer-free woman with the strong family history of breast cancer associated with a mutation of BRCA 1 tests positive, what is she to do? With a lifetime risk of 85 per cent of developing breast cancer she may consider prophylactic mastectomies. As well, she could consider removal of the ovaries since the gene mutation is also associated with an increased risk of ovarian cancer. There may also be a slightly increased risk of bowel cancer which may at least warrant screening. Alternatively, she may decide to undergo intense screening to detect any breast cancers early and not have a mastectomy straight away. The point is that she should be aware of these possibilities before being tested, since the result may have a profound influence on her life and psychological wellbeing.

There are general bioethical considerations to genetic testing. Individuals should be counselled and give their consent. The result may disclose information about other relatives which they may not wish to know. Test results should be confidential, but in the future such testing could affect insurance status and results be demanded for that reason.

Genetic counselling clinics will be in increasing demand as the genetic basis for more cancers becomes known.

SUMMARY

The best evidence for the efficacy of population-based screening is found for breast cancer and cancer of the cervix. It is currently recommended that women 50 years and above have routine mammograms with clinical breast examinations. Regular cervical smear tests should begin when a woman becomes sexually active and continue into old age. Screening for cancer of the large bowel with faecal occult blood tests reduces mortality from large bowel cancer. Patients with positive tests proceed to colonoscopy. Routine testing for prostate cancer is problematic because of difficulties in assessing its impact on a disease that is not always fatal, and not knowing how best to treat early disease. Public education programs to increase the awareness of detecting melanomas early seem sensible but their impact is difficult to quantify. There is insufficient evidence to warrant population screening for other cancers. Genetic screening to assess an individual's risk of developing cancer when there is a family history must be preceded by appropriate counselling.

5

How do you treat cancer?

The value of a principle is the number of things it will explain; and there is no good theory of disease which does not at once suggest a cure.

—*Ralph Waldo Emerson*

I would like to start on a positive note. Bernard Baruch once said: 'There are no such things as incurables; there are only things for which man has not found a cure.' If this is true and we keep looking we will develop better treatments and begin to cure more types of cancer, even when they are widespread. One of the reasons that Chapter 1 concentrates on the mechanisms of the development of cancer is that they do suggest, as Emerson contends, possible cures. Often, however, things are more complex than a theory suggests and what will work in a test-tube is ineffective in the complex environment of the human body.

If cancers are detected before they spread, they may be curable with local treatments. Surgery has been the mainstay of this approach. Radiotherapy can also cure local tumours which are small enough to be encompassed in a treatment area.

If a cancer has spread beyond the site where it started to grow it will need a treatment that I refer to as a systemic treatment, since it needs to circulate throughout the whole body system. Giving drugs (chemotherapy) that will circulate throughout the body in the bloodstream would be one example. Other examples we look at include immunotherapy, which tries to use the body's immune system against cancer cells, biological therapy, which uses substances found to be produced by the body as treatments, and the emerging gene therapies.

SURGERY FOR CANCER

Surgery for cancer is an ancient treatment. The Edwin Smith papyrus from ancient Egypt, dated about the seventeenth century BC, discusses surgery from the head down to the middle of the chest and includes removal of tumours. In the early nineteenth century a large tumour of the ovary was successfully removed from a woman in America by MacDowell. Many surgeons became famous for describing surgical techniques for treating various cancers. An example is William Halsted who in 1890 described the radical mastectomy as a treatment for breast cancer. This technique removes the breast and surrounding tissues *en bloc*. Halsted is also credited with introducing rubber gloves into operations, not initially for himself but, in a demonstration that chivalry was not dead, to protect the hands of his operating nurse, whom he later married. The story also serves to remind us that the successes of early surgical procedures were also due to the evolution of the related disciplines of infection control and anaesthesia.

Cancer surgery has had to evolve in line with changing knowledge about the spread of cancer. For example, the Halsted mastectomy was developed under the assumption that extensive local surgery would cure breast cancer because there was an orderly progression of the cancer from the breast to the lymph glands that drained the breast and then to more distant sites. The procedure is no longer used because it is now recognised that small groups of cells can spread beyond the initial site very early in the development of the cancer. The reason that cancer returns after extensive surgery is that it is estimated that seven of every ten people with solid cancers have microscopic spread beyond the primary site when they first present, even though it can't be detected. Most of the deaths from cancer will be from the distant spread.

There is no point in doing extremely extensive and disfiguring local surgery in the hope that it will improve the cure rate. Instead, the surgery is modified so that it removes all the local cancer which can be seen. This may be curative in some early cancers, as is apparent from the success of the breast screening program. A wider local area can be sterilised with radiation therapy. In other cases, additional systemic treatment is added to surgery to deal with the more widespread cells.

I tell patients who wonder why a surgical approach is not being considered for their cancers that there is no survival benefit to cutting out part of a tumour; you may as well not remove any of it and save yourself the side effects of surgery. In general, a surgical approach to curing cancer is only used if there is a reasonable chance that *all* the cancer can be removed. There are many roles for surgery in the treatment of cancer, ranging from prevention through curative treatment to palliation, or control of symptoms.

Surgery for the prevention of cancer

There are many conditions that identify individuals with a high risk of developing cancer. We have discussed familial polyposis coli where almost all patients will develop bowel cancer during their lifetime. To prevent this, most patients undergo preventive removal of the large bowel before they are twenty years old. More controversial is the removal of both breasts and ovaries in patients who have a family history of breast cancer and carry the same gene mutation as the family member who presented with the breast cancer (see Chapter 4).

Surgery to diagnose and stage cancer

Biopsies of cancers can range from placing a needle into the cancer to obtain a few cells to opening an abdomen to obtain a piece of a tumour. The preferred techniques are the least invasive needle biopsies but sometimes when the pattern of a cancer is important, as is the case with cancers of lymph glands, then a whole lump may need to be removed. Biopsies can also be done under direct vision through an endoscope, which can enter body cavities without large cuts, but there is a limitation to the size of the samples that can be recovered.

Of historical interest is the use of the staging laparotomy for Hodgkin's disease. This involved opening the abdomen and sampling various lymph nodes and removing the spleen to gauge the extent of the spread of the disease so that appropriate treatment could be planned. If you knew the disease was localised to a group of lymph glands, radiotherapy was an option; otherwise, chemotherapy was required. The advent of CT scans which imaged the contents of the abdomen replaced the need for surgical staging.

Surgery to treat cancer

For many cancers the surgeon is responsible for local control of the tumour. The importance of the likelihood of cure determining the extent of surgery can be illustrated by the treatment of a few common cancers. Early melanomas can be cured by surgery. The likelihood of cure depends on the depth of penetration of the melanoma. Traditionally, melanomas were removed with wide margins of normal tissue of at least 5 centimetres. Recently, the margins have been reduced because it was not the margin but the depth of penetration that was determining the outcome; what was required surgically was that all the melanoma was removed. This has meant that fewer defects have needed skin grafts.

Early breast cancer that is small and confined to the breast can be cured by surgery alone. The chances of curing larger breast cancers with spread to lymph glands under the arm are less. Removal of the lymph glands under the arm gives information about the likelihood of survival; it depends on the number involved and is part of local regional control of the cancer. It can also help to determine what additional treatment is needed, although this can now be planned independently of this information. Local control, however, is not the arbiter of survival, so extensive surgery offers limited benefit. Also, local control need not be achieved with surgery alone. It has been found that just removing the cancerous lump and irradiating the rest of the breast gives similar outcomes to a mastectomy but obviously leaves the breast intact for a better cosmetic outcome.

Cancer of the large bowel that is confined to the bowel wall has a high chance of cure if it is adequately surgically removed. The main treatment for sarcomas—cancers of structural tissues such as muscles and bones—is surgery. Similarly, some thyroid cancers can be surgically cured.

Surgery may involve burning the cancer. This occurs with superficial bladder cancers where the inside of the bladder is seen through a cystoscope and suspicious areas are destroyed. In the same way, lasers may be used to destroy cancers in the airways.

A different role for surgery in cancers that can't be completely removed is to remove at least the bulk of the cancer. This seems to contradict my statement about the futility of removing only part of a tumour. The concept relies on having a very effective treatment for the rest of the disease. Debulking surgery for cancer of the ovary, followed by chemotherapy, falls into this category.

Surgery for metastatic cancer

Some cancers have only a few metastases and they can be removed surgically. An isolated metastasis to the brain with no other disease is one example. It is possible to remove a few metastases from the liver when it is the only site of spread. If the primary site is large bowel cancer and there is a single metastasis in the liver, 25 per cent of patients can expect to be cured. Lung metastases may also be removed if they are unresponsive to drug therapy.

Another different role for surgery in widespread disease is to manipulate hormones for those cancers that are sensitive to hormones. The two leading examples would be removal of the testicles to withdraw the male hormone stimulus in prostate cancer, and removing the ovaries in women with breast cancer to reduce the stimulus from female hormones.

Organ transplants in cancer

It is tempting to ask why an organ invaded by cancer can't simply be removed and replaced with a transplanted organ. Liver transplants could be one example. In general, you will realise that you know the answer. There would be no point to removing an organ containing secondaries since the primary could send out more metastases. For a primary, the only possibility would be the replacement of a liver which contained a small primary cancer where you could be absolutely sure that no secondary spread had occurred. In other cases, a large operation would be quickly followed by the return of the disease.

Surgery for symptom control

Surgery can be part of palliating the symptoms of cancer. Painful fractures of bones that have been eroded by cancer may require stabilising by the surgical insertion of pins or plates. A bowel cancer may be partially blocking the bowel and causing spasms of pain in the abdomen. This can be relieved by removing the affected bowel or by creating a colostomy where the bowel contents drain externally into a bag on the wall of the abdomen before they reach the site of obstruction by the cancer. A kidney cancer that is painful because it is big, or is responsible for continual bleeding into the urine, can be removed to alleviate those symptoms. Obstructions to hollow tubes in the body such as airways or the oesophagus can be managed by stents or laser treatment.

Complications of surgery

The risks of a surgical procedure, particularly if it is for palliation, must be carefully weighed against the likely outcome. Risks associated with surgery include anaesthetic risks and the chance of forming blood clots through prolonged immobilisation. The main complications of surgery centre on post-operative bleeding or infection. Most of these can be anticipated and treated but are still particular problems in the very sick or elderly patient.

RADIATION THERAPY

The second of the treatments to deal with localised cancer is radiotherapy. X-rays were discovered by Wilhelm Roentgen in 1895. The following year Antonie Becquerel and Marie Curie discovered the radioactive properties of uranium and radium. In early 1896, E.H. Grubbe described the first use of radiation as a therapy in Chicago when he irradiated Mrs Rose Lee's breast. The effects of radiation on normal tissues became apparent within months of the development of x-rays, when a radiation worker reported hair loss.

Radiotherapy can be used to cure localised cancers or to shrink them as part of controlling any symptoms they may be causing. To understand why radiotherapy is delivered in the way that it is, you must first realise that the goal is to give the cancer the maximum dose while trying to spare as much of the normal tissue around it as possible. I refer to it as 'a local therapy' because, in general, all the benefit and the side effects will occur in the radiation field—that is, the area being irradiated.

Both the size of the field and the dose are limited by the effects on normal tissues. Normal tissues will tolerate a certain dose of radiation before breaking down. This varies for each type of tissue. Also, once that maximum dose has been given to a particular area, no further radiation can ever be given to that area without the risk of normal tissue breakdown. The damage accumulates with each radiotherapy dose and causes permanent changes to the tissues and their blood supply.

How does radiation kill cancer?

Radiation for therapy is either x-rays produced by electrical machines called linear accelerators or gamma rays produced by the decay of radioactive isotopes such as cobalt. The radiation used in therapy is of very short wavelength. When an x-ray hits an atom or molecule in a cell it knocks off one of its electrons, forming unstable ions which can damage cells (hence the term 'ionising radiation'). As the x-ray beam passes through tissues it will randomly ionise cells in its path. Sometimes, it will hit the nucleus of a cell and sometimes the surrounding cytoplasm, or even the tissue outside the cell. The major target of radiation for cell killing is the DNA, but damage to other vital structures in the cell can also kill it by the indirect effect of the short-lived ions produced by the radiation. The important principle in killing a cell is to stop it dividing.

There is an old saying that a cancer cell doesn't know it is dead until it tries to divide. This is fairly accurate and explains the delay between delivering the radiation and seeing a tumour shrink. Radiation can kill rapidly by turning on the program that leads to programmed cell death (apoptosis). Often, however, it doesn't kill the cell until the cell tries to divide, when the damage to the DNA will prevent this happening. In the meantime, the cell can remain functional. The cell may divide but produce sterile or abnormal offspring. The cell is most sensitive to radiation during the phase when the DNA strands are separating so that division into daughter cells can take place.

Not all the cells damaged by radiation die. Repair of the damage can occur, particularly after a low dose. Some cells are more resistant to radiation. Cells that are deprived of oxygen, such as those in the centre of a rapidly growing cancer, can be far more resistant than well oxygenated cells, for example. This gives us an insight into research directions in radiotherapy. Attempts are being made to combine radiation with drugs that can sensitise cells to radiation, and sensitise oxygen-starved cells. Some chemotherapy drugs increase the efficacy of radiation either by sensitising cells to it, preventing any repair taking place, or just adding one way of killing to another.

Limiting damage to normal cells

Radiotherapy is not specific to cancer. It will kill normal cells in its path as well. To maximise the benefit of radiotherapy we need to minimise the damage to normal tissues while ensuring the tumour is killed. The energy of the radiation will determine at what depth of penetration of the body it will cause most damage. The size of the radiation field and what tissues are in it will determine what dose can be tolerated. Fractionating the radiotherapy (i.e. giving multiple small doses instead of one large dose) is important in achieving the balance between damage to the tumour and damage to normal tissues.

Radiotherapy is given over a block of time, often five days each week for several weeks if curative doses are to be given. You can vary the dose per daily fraction, the number of fractions or the time over which the fractions are delivered. The more immediate damage to tissues will depend on the time over which the therapy is given. Later damage to normal tissues is more dependent on the total dose given and the size of each fraction. The clinical effect of fractionated radiotherapy will depend on how much repair of either the tumour or normal tissues can occur between fractions. Also, both normal tissues and tumour can be repopulated with cells between fractions. As we saw in Chapter 1, growth may increase as a tumour shrinks and the repopulation may be accelerated by treatment.

Current research into more effective ways of delivering radiotherapy exploit these observations. Hyperfractionation means giving multiple smaller fractions within a day. Accelerated fractionation is giving normal-sized fractions but more than once a day. Six hours between fractions may allow damage repair, which is certainly desirable in normal tissues, but is too short for any repopulation. Encouraging results have been obtained. Accelerating the fractionation would certainly make sense in rapidly growing tumours where quite significant growth could occur between fractions if they are given once each day.

Maximising the dose to the tumour and sparing normal tissues is the goal of planning radiotherapy fields. Using CT scans and computers, the various doses that the tumour and surrounding tissue will receive can be calculated. These are displayed rather like weather maps but showing dose distribution instead of lines of equal atmospheric pressure. Dose distribution maps can become quite complex—rather than simply delivering a dose of radiotherapy to a single field from the front, back or sides, multiple beams can be angled to intersect over the tumour, sparing vital structures such as the spinal cord. Three-dimensional planning is necessary to encompass the whole volume of the cancer.

When delivering radiotherapy, part of the target can be shielded to protect normal tissue. If you place lead blocks at the point of exit of the x-ray beam, it will not pass through them, and you can imagine a shadow being cast on the target tissue below. When irradiating the lymph glands in the chest you may wish to shield the lungs in this way. Such shielding can be tailored for each patient and its positioning can be checked by x-ray pictures taken in the treatment position during a course of treatment.

When do we use radiotherapy?

Radiotherapy can be given in large doses in an attempt to cure a localised cancer. It can be used alone or with other treatments to cure some cancers including lymphomas, head and neck cancers, skin cancers, lower bowel cancers, breast cancers, lung cancers, oesophageal cancers, bladder cancers and genital organ cancers in men and women. For symptom control, or palliation, radiation can be very effective for controlling radiosensitive tumours that are blocking airways, pressing on nerves, bleeding or causing pain. Bone pain in particular responds very well to radiotherapy.

The side effects of radiotherapy

Although there are total-body and half-body techniques where low doses are delivered to wide areas for specific purposes such as obliterating the bone marrow prior to transplantation, or palliating widespread bone pain, most radiotherapy is given to localised areas. This means that the side effects will depend on the tissues irradiated and be confined to the area of the body receiving the radiation. The damage to tissues tends to accumulate with each fraction of radiotherapy. The acute effects will occur towards the end of the course of therapy and resolve within days to weeks. More important are the late effects which signify more permanent tissue damage. It is the late effects that may be avoided by altering the fractionation schedule. Let us look at what side effects you may expect from irradiating various tissues.

Skin

Skin reactions occur when tumours near to the skin surface are irradiated. An example would be radiotherapy for breast cancer. With higher-energy irradiation the peak dose is well beneath the skin and so skin reactions are less common if deep-seated cancers are being irradiated. The immediate or acute reaction occurring towards the end of a course of radiation is a redness of the skin followed by itchy dry skin peeling or, if more severe, weeping ulcerated skin like a very bad sunburn. This will heal just like a sunburn and creams can be used to control the discomfort. If there is any hair in the field, hair loss will occur, and the sweat glands may dry up in the area treated. If there are late effects, these will include tanning or loss of pigmentation of the skin, a woodiness of the skin and the appearance of multiple small blood vessels just under the skin. The skin may remain more sensitive to sun exposure. With severely affected skin, ulceration and difficulty in healing when cut can occur, because of damage to the skin's blood supply.

Mouth and bowel

Similar burning side effects are the acute side effects in other areas. There is loss of taste, and mouth ulcers and dryness in the mouth occur. Mouthwashes for symptom control can be used until healing occurs. Dry mouth is often a long-term result of radiation to the mouth. Dental work, particularly extractions, should be done prior to radiotherapy with time for healing, to prevent permanent damage to the jaw-bones.

Lower down, if the oesophagus is irradiated, patients will experience pain on swallowing. If the stomach and small bowel are in the field of irradiation, nausea and vomiting may result. Inflammation of the large bowel may result in pain, bleeding and diarrhoea. All acute effects should reverse within a couple of weeks but it can be a serious problem if these are late effects, indicating more profound tissue damage.

Brain and spinal cord

Above a certain radiation dose, damage to the brain or spinal cord is likely. This is called the tissue's tolerance to radiation. The tolerance level is well known and radiation is planned not to exceed this dose. Acute side effects include a somnolence syndrome six weeks after irradiation of the brain, particularly in children, when patients feel excessively sleepy for a couple of weeks, and then recover. After spinal cord irradiation, some patients experience temporary shooting sensations down the body when bending the neck. Late effects in these tissues—which actually result from permanent damage to the nervous system tissues—may cause symptoms that mimic having a brain tumour or a cancer pressing on the spinal cord.

Other late effects may depend on what other organs are irradiated. If the lens of the eye receives too high a dose when irradiating the brain, cataracts will develop. Late endocrine problems can be caused by irradiation of the pituitary gland at the base of the brain because of the decreased hormone output from the gland. A similar picture is seen with late occurrence of an underactive thyroid after irradiation of the neck.

Other organs

I have chosen specific examples and there is no need to review each organ system in detail. You can see that normal tissue tolerance limits the size of the possible fields, which is why radiotherapy is a local treatment. You can't irradiate lung without causing scarring and therefore the amount of lung in a field must be limited. The heart may be inflamed by radiation or its blood supply damaged, thus accelerating coronary artery disease. Too much bone marrow in a field will cause low blood counts, a side effect that is discussed in more detail with chemotherapy (Chapter 5). Irradiating bones in children can prevent the bones from growing, causing deformities in adulthood. It requires only small doses of radiotherapy to the testes or ovaries to cause infertility, but this is variable. Radiation can be used instead of surgery if ablation of the ovaries is required as part of the hormonal treatment of breast cancer.

Second cancers as a late effect

Although uncommon, it is ironic that second cancers can be late effects of radiation therapy. They occur several years after the therapy. In general, the possibility of developing second cancers does not alter the decision to use radiotherapy—if the original cancer is not cured the patient will not live long enough to develop a second cancer. Much of what we know of second cancers has come from the successful treatment of lymphomas and the follow-up of victims of radiation exposure from nuclear weapons and nuclear accidents. The most common cancers to occur after radiation are leukaemias, cancers of the thyroid gland, and cancers of soft tissue and bone which usually occur within the radiation field. These second cancers have to be treated on their merits, although usually no further radiation can be used in a previously irradiated area. The thyroid gland is very sensitive to being irradiated, but can also take up and concentrate the radioactive iodine produced after radiation exposure. This is why, after the Chernobyl nuclear reactor accident in 1986, Europeans were taking iodine so that their thyroids were flooded with iodine before the nuclear cloud passed over.

What happens when you need radiotherapy?

Radiation oncologists often work as part of a multidisciplinary team. If radiotherapy is the treatment of choice you will have the x-rays and scans that allow planning of the radiation fields. With the aid of computers, the best configuration of fields to give the appropriate dose for the tumour volume (while sparing as much of the normal tissue as possible) will be calculated.

The next step is a visit to the simulator. This machine mimics a radiation treatment machine and is used to line up the patient into the correct position for treatment. The same position will need to be adopted for each fraction of radiotherapy. Lining up may involve using laser lights to position the patient, using markers on the skin or bony landmarks, or checking the position with x-rays. For some areas, such as the head and neck, a mould may be made to create a clear mask which is worn to keep the head still and in exactly the same position each time. As mentioned above, lead shielding in the head of the machine may be added to spare normal tissues; the position of this is checked by taking x-rays on the simulator when the patient is placed in the treatment position. These preparations ensure that patients can be quickly placed in the correct treatment position each time they reach the treatment machine.

The treatment machine is often a linear accelerator these days and consists of a couch around which the x-ray head can rotate, so that it can treat from different angles according to what fields are planned. It is in a room with heavy concrete and lead shielding. The patient is left alone in the room while being irradiated but is monitored with video cameras from the control room. Each fraction of therapy may take only a few seconds to give. The patient does not feel anything. It is just like having an x-ray. If curative treatment is planned, the therapy may be given every weekday for six or seven weeks. No acute side effects may occur until the last week or two of the treatment. For palliative therapy, as little as one dose may be all that is required.

Special types of radiotherapy

In some special circumstances, radiotherapy can be delivered continuously by radiotherapy sources implanted into tumours using thin wires, or sources loaded into applicators passed into body cavities. A good example is the treatment of cancer of the cervix. Here sources can be placed very close to the cervix and left in place for many hours. This can be combined with external beam radiotherapy as part of radical treatment.

Sometimes a radioactive isotope can be injected. The ability of thyroid tissue to take up radioactive iodine can be used in the treatment of widespread thyroid cancer. Radioactive iodine is injected into the thyroid tissue and the tissue is ablated by the dose of radiotherapy it receives.

Stereotactic radiosurgery is a clever technique where small deep-seated brain tumours that would be impossible to reach surgically can be treated with radiotherapy directed to the target tumour by CT scan. The skull is immobilised in a frame and a high dose of radiation delivered precisely to the cancer, thereby sparing most of the surrounding normal brain.

Finally, the characteristics of the particle used influence the outcome. The use of heavy particles such as neutrons, instead of the photons and electrons that are used in conventional therapy, may allow improved dose distribution and help over-come the problems created by oxygen lack. It takes complex equipment to generate neutrons and their use is still confined to experiments in a few centres.

Radiotherapy combined with other treatments

Radiotherapy can be combined with other treatments to improve the outcome. Later in this chapter I discuss some indications for using various treatment modalities in sequence. Some treatments are designed to be used with radiotherapy. Certain drugs sensitise normal cells to radiation, others sensitise oxygen-starved cells to radiation or protect normal tissue from the effects of radiation, and all these are the subject of research designed to increase the efficacy of radiotherapy. The goal of many of these treatments is to increase the effect of the radio-therapy on the cancer over the effect it has on normal tissues. Locally heating a cancer and then irradiating it is another ongoing area of research. We look at the combined effects of radiotherapy and chemotherapy after the next section.

CHEMOTHERAPY FOR CANCER

Chemotherapy, or drug therapy, is used to treat cancers which are known to have spread beyond the primary site, or as an addition to local treatment if there is a high probability that microscopic metastases have occurred. The drugs are often called cytotoxic drugs, which simply means they are toxic to cells. There is a stereotype that chemotherapy is nasty and this belief causes unnecessary anxiety. The stereotype is perhaps fuelled by the Hollywood portrayal of the heroine diagnosed with cancer and treated with chemotherapy who loses her hair, wastes away and dies anyway. This is simply not the usual case.

People must realise that different chemotherapy is used for different cancers and it is a case of 'horses for courses'. More aggressive chemotherapy may be warranted when cure is the aim, whereas less toxicity is acceptable if the aim is to palliate symptoms. Almost all the side effects of chemotherapy are temporary and reversible, and the decision to give chemotherapy is always a balance between the potential outcome and side effects. The treatment is not allowed to be worse than the disease. Temporary side effects need to be balanced by the longer-term benefits of control of the cancer.

Most people associate chemotherapy with injections into the veins and are surprised to learn that some of the drugs are available as tablets. Irrespective of the route of administration, the drugs enter the bloodstream and can circulate to wherever the tumour has spread.

The word 'chemotherapy' was first used by Paul Ehrlich in the early 1900s to describe the use of known chemicals to treat infections by parasites. He studied the effect of the drugs on infectious diseases in laboratory animals. George Clowes subsequently developed a method of transplanting tumours into rodents to enable systematic testing of anti-cancer chemotherapy drugs.

Reports of drugs being used for widespread cancer date from the first century. Colchicine from the chinchona tree was tried as an anti-cancer drug. Heavy metals were used to treat skin cancers and arsenic achieved some success with chronic myeloid leukaemia. The first scientific development of anti-cancer drugs came from the use of alkylating agents such as nitrogen mustard gas as a weapon of war. Sulphur mustard gas was used in the First World War.

During the Second World War, nitrogen mustard was tested in animals bearing lymphomas by a team including Goodman and Gilman at Yale. The use of these agents in humans was said to have been accelerated after Allied ships were bombed in an Italian port during the Second World War. Some of the ships were carrying nitrogen mustard gas which spread around the harbour. Colonel S.F. Alexander, who cared for the casualties, reported the effect of the gas in suppressing the bone marrow, blood counts and lymphoid tissues of the sufferers. Nitrogen mustard, a derivative of the gas, was used to treat six patients with lymphomas, including Hodgkin's disease, at Yale in 1943, with shrinkage of the disease. Due to the secrecy of the war gas program, the results were not reported until 1946.

In 1944 it was observed that a vitamin, folic acid, helped leukaemic cells (malignant white blood cells) to grow. Drugs that blocked folate were developed and the first successful treatment of leukaemia with these drugs was reported in 1948. As more drugs were developed, the next step was to treat cancers with combinations of cytotoxic drugs; in the 1960s, cures of Hodgkin's disease and childhood leukaemias with drug combinations were reported. The search for new drugs and combinations continues. Different types of drugs kill the cancer cells in different ways.

How do drugs kill cancer?

Most of the drugs that we use today disrupt the DNA in cells and, thus, kill cells when they try to divide. It must be understood that chemotherapy does not target cancer cells specifically. It will also kill dividing cells in normal tissues, which helps explain many of the side effects of the drugs. The normal tissues are often better at repairing themselves between chemo-therapy courses than the cancer. The other reason that cancers are more sensitive to chemotherapy is that a higher proportion of a cancer is actively dividing than is the case for normal tissues.

Drugs are classified by how and where they act (see Table 5.1). If we first consider nitrogen mustard we find that it falls into a class of drugs called alkylating agents.

They act by bonding to the bases of the DNA chains. This can cause the two strands of DNA, which are wound around each other, to be linked together, or breaks in the strands to occur. This will obviously affect the strands dividing and being copied. The bonding to the strands can occur whether the cell is dividing or not and at any time in the dividing process, but will usually only kill a cell that tries to divide.

Another class of drugs is known as antimetabolites. These are substances that bear a resemblance to naturally occurring substances and can be substituted for them; but they don't have the same function and so the cell grinds to a halt. For example, methotrexate can substitute for folic acid and stop the building blocks of DNA being produced. The drug 5 fluorouracil, among other things, can substitute for one of the bases in RNA and interfere with its function. In general, it does not matter which part of the dividing cycle the cell is in for these drugs to be effective.

Antitumour antibiotics are isolated from bacteria. They disrupt DNA by slipping between its chains and preventing division. Doxorubicin is a common example of this class of drugs and is particularly noted by patients because of its red colour. Bleomycin is another example of this class.

There is a series of drugs derived from plants. Vincristine and vinblastine from the periwinkle plant act at the site of the spindle that forms to enable the duplicated DNA to separate so that two daughter cells can be formed with identical copies (see Chapter 1). These drugs stop the microtubules which make up the spindle from joining together. Only cells at this specific phase of the cycle of division can be affected by these drugs.

Table 5.1 Common chemotherapy drugs

Alkylating agents	Drugs from plants
Nitrogen mustard	Vincristine
Cyclophosphamide	Vinblastine
Ifosfamide	Vindesine
Melphalan	Etoposide
Chlorambucil	Teniposide
Busulphan	Paclitaxel
Lomustine	Docetaxel
Carmustine	Irinotecan
Dacarbazine	Topotecan
Thiotepin	
Hexamethylmelamine	
Antimetabolites	**Miscellaneous**
Methotrexate	Cisplatin
Fluorouracil	Carboplatin
Mercaptopurine	L-Asparaginase
Fludarabine phosphate	Hydroxyurea
Thioguanine	Procarbazine
Cytosine arabinoside	Mitotane
	Amsacrine
	Mitoxantrone
Antitumour antibiotics	
Daunorubicin	
Doxorubicin	
Idarubicin	
Epirubicin	
Actinomycin-D	
Mitomycin	
Bleomycin	

More recently, drugs derived from the bark and needles of yew trees, paclitaxel and docetaxel, were also found to act at the spindle but with the opposite effect—they allow the spindle to form but not to disassemble.

Drugs derived from modified substances from the mandrake plant, the podophyllotoxins etoposide and teniposide, are also specific for a phase of the cell's division cycle, stopping it before the spindle forms. These drugs can cause breaks in the DNA by affecting the way the DNA is folded.

Finally, there are several drugs that come from a variety of sources and fit into no particular group. Examples include the drug cisplatin, a metal salt that binds to DNA, asparaginase derived from bacteria that interferes in tumour cells with the making of proteins, and procarbazine with a structure similar to that of drugs used to treat depression which breaks down into substances that damage DNA.

New drug research is focusing increasingly on the development of drugs which have targets other than DNA. For example, some of the growth factor receptors in the cell membrane could be targeted. Proteins in the cell that signal oncogenes or are involved in the initiation of programmed cell death will, in theory, be useful targets. Other research focuses on developing effective chemotherapy with fewer side effects.

Where do cytotoxic drugs come from?

Although 'a cabbage patch' may be a flippant answer to the question of the origin of cytotoxics, it may not be as far off as it sounds. Some drugs are discovered by accident, some were purpose-built in the laboratory and others have been found in various plants and animals, although not as yet cabbages.

Accidents will happen

Discovery of important treatments by chance observation has a long history in medicine. This occurred with the cytotoxic drug, cisplatin, which forms the backbone for the very successful treatment of testicular and ovarian cancers, and head and neck, lung and bladder cancers, among others. In the mid 1960s, Barnett Rosenberg was studying the effect of electric fields on the growth of bacteria in culture. He designed an experiment where he placed bacteria into a nutrient solution and passed an electric current through it between two electrodes made of platinum. When he did this he observed that the growth rate of the bacteria was lessened and their pattern of growth altered. This was attributed to the formation of platinum complexes due to platinum dissolving from the electrodes and forming complexes with elements in the nutrient. As a result of this observation, neutral platinum complexes were discovered to have a selective effect on rapidly dividing bacteria and so they were tested on cancer. Cisplatin was found to have substantial anti-cancer activity.

The vinca alkaloids were found to be anti-cancer drugs only after the periwinkle plant from which they come was screened for anti-diabetic activity.

Designer cytotoxic drugs

In the laboratory, drugs can be designed to carry out various functions. Sometimes, drugs can be designed from scratch to disrupt a specific target. If you know, for example, that one way of disrupting DNA is for a drug with two arms to slide between the folds of DNA, it may be beneficial to design a drug with three arms to see if this is more effective. Alternatively, if you know that cisplatin is effective but has serious side effects (such as the potential for damaging the kidney), you may see if substituting other chemicals for those attached to the central platinum in cisplatin will change that. A large number of close relatives, or analogues, of cisplatin have been produced. Carboplatin is one that is routinely used; it has a different pattern of side effects with less kidney toxicity but more bone marrow suppression.

A drug used for some other purpose may be adapted for use against cancers. Mitotane is related to the insecticide DDT and causes shrinkage of the adrenal gland; not surprisingly, it is used in adrenal carcinoma.

The other way of designing new drugs and making them in the laboratory is to try to copy some of the complex chemicals in nature that have been found to be cytotoxic. Making them in the laboratory ensures a more plentiful supply and they can also be altered, as described above, to see if more potent drugs with less toxicity can be created.

Chemotherapy from nature

In a world where there is much talk of natural therapies it is sobering to realise how many chemotherapy drugs come from plants, animals and bacteria. In their native form, however, they are associated with other substances and possible toxic impurities that are unwanted. We therefore extract the drug we want and purify it before giving it to patients.

Some examples of drugs from nature were given above. There were the vinca alkaloids from the periwinkle plant (*Vinca rosea Linn*), the podophyllotoxins from the American mandrake (*Podophyllin peltatum*) and the taxanes from the Western yew and European yews (*Taxus brevifolia*). More recently, the drugs topotecan and irinotecan are being developed. They are derived from a northern Chinese tree (*Camptotheca acuminata*).

We also have drugs that are isolated from bacteria—the antitumour antibiotics are isolated from the culture broth of streptomyces, and L-asparaginase is isolated from bacteria, commonly *Escherichia coli*.

The undersea world has also been explored for new drugs. The first success was in the derivation of drugs from the Caribbean sponge (*Tetha crypta*). Today cytosine arabinoside is an important drug in curing acute leukaemia. More bounty from the Caribbean is the sea squirt (*Trididemnum solidum*) which gives rise to didemnin B, a drug in current trials. The bryostatins are being tested after being isolated from a marine bryozoan(*Bugula neitina*) found growing on the bottoms of ships in harbours.

You may wonder why the sea, or indeed a forest, should be a source of cytotoxic drugs. We could speculate that, in the crowded environment of the sea floor or forest, it may be of survival advantage to have a toxin in your bark or shell to protect yourself from attack, or perhaps to poison the next-door neighbour. A large number of plant and animal extracts, which could possess anti-cancer activity because they have the ability to kill cells, are stored and await testing.

Testing potential anti-cancer drugs

There is a long process for testing new drugs that starts off in the laboratory, passes through an animal testing stage and ends up with clinical trials. The largest screening effort for new anti-cancer drugs is mounted by the National Cancer Institute in the United States.

Initial screening of drugs

Until the mid 1980s, the screening of new chemicals for anti-cancer activity involved initial testing against leukaemia cells from mice in the laboratory. If the drugs were active they went on to the next screen, consisting of mouse and human tumours transplanted into mice. The problem with this system is that it failed to find agents that were active in the common solid cancers. It repeatedly identified drugs that were useful in lymphomas and leukaemias. How the drugs worked was not defined by this method of screening.

The current system involves cancer cells from humans including lung, bowel, melanoma, kidney, ovary, brain, leukaemia and breast cancers, selected because of known patterns of response to drugs, dependence on growth factors or known expression of oncogenes, so that these characteristics of solid cancers can be targeted. Furthermore, if you use large numbers, say 60 cell lines, you can build up a characteristic pattern of response for each drug where new agents can be compared with established agents and the most novel active agents prioritised for further testing. A clue about the mechanism of action is also obtained, depending on which cell lines the new drug is able to kill.

The human cell line that is most sensitive to the drug being tested is then tested as a graft into a mouse. The drug can then be tested for its antitumour effect in a living animal. If it is not as effective as it was in cell culture, there may be something about the way it is broken down or distributed in the animal that is preventing it from being effective. It may be possible to deal with this by making further changes to the structure of the drug.

Drugs are usually tested first in small animals such as mice and rats. Then larger animals such as dogs are used to find out how it is taken up by the body, how long it circulates in the bloodstream, how it is processed and how it is expelled from the body. The same small and large animals are used to test how toxic the drug is to the various body organs at various doses. This provides information on how to use the drug in the first human studies.

Phase I, II, III clinical testing of new drugs

Clinical testing proceeds in a stepwise fashion with several types of trials. The initial studies, or phase I studies, are designed to find the maximum tolerated dose of the new drug and what side effects will occur. The aim of these trials is to find the optimum dose for testing the efficacy of the drug. Starting at a dose considered safe, based on the animal studies, groups of three patients are treated. If there are no severe side effects the next group is treated at a higher dose and so on until a side effect is seen, which will limit further dose escalation. (For the mathematicians among you, the dose escalation scheme is usually a modified Fibonacci series.) The dose for the next phase of testing will be the dose level immediately below that at which the dose-limiting toxicity was seen.

Which patients enter a phase I study? The usual candidates are those patients whose cancers have failed to respond to, or have relapsed following, conventional chemotherapy or for which no standard chemotherapy exists. There is no guarantee of success in these studies, since this represents the earliest testing of a drug in humans. Yet our currently active drugs were once the subject of phase I trials and responses were seen, so it is the hope of investigators and patients alike that some individual will benefit. If there is no response, the patient will not remain on the drug. Even then, some patients gain satisfaction from being able to contribute to a study focused on improving the wellbeing of future patients with cancer. It is this aspect of participating in a carefully conducted scientific study of an unproven drug that elevates it above trying the unproven remedies offered by snake oil salesmen.

Phase II trials are designed to test the effectiveness of a drug against a specific cancer type, to see if it has sufficient activity to warrant further testing in comparison with the current standard treatment. The dose and schedule identified from the phase I study are used in testing the drug against specific cancers. A reasonable idea of the response rate can be obtained with 30 or 40 patients, but only those cancers where there is no effective treatment can be treated with the experimental drug as the first line of treatment. Occasionally, a clue to what tumour type will respond can be found during the phase I trial. However, many of the patients in a phase I trial will have received less than the optimal dose if they are early participants and are treated at the lower dose levels, and many different types of cancer will be represented in the trial, so that often no responses are seen until the phase II program.

It is important to know what an oncologist defines as a response. A complete response, as it suggests, is complete disappearance of the cancer. The treatment will often be continued for further courses after this point because we know there is still microscopic disease left after we can no longer see it on scans or feel it. We also describe a partial response. So that we can compare the activity of a drug when used by doctors in one hospital with results from another hospital, the agreed definition of a partial response is shrinkage of the tumour by at least 50 per cent. Since there is still cancer present, a partial response may not improve survival, but shrinking the cancer that much should control any symptoms it is causing. Any lesser shrinkage is usually not counted as a response.

Phase II studies may also uncover further side effects and patients are followed to see the duration of the response and the survival. It is on the basis of all these endpoints that a decision is made whether to continue development of the drug.

Phase III trials test the new drug against the standard treatment in a randomised trial. This means that patients are allocated by chance to one treatment or the other. This eliminates any chance of bias—such as only the fit patients being selected for the experimental treatment. If there are enough patients, any factors other than the treatment that may impact on the outcome should be evenly distributed between the two treatment groups. Such factors may include age, sex, extent of the cancer and how fit the patient is. A randomised design means that the circumstance in which the treatment is given is the same for both groups, eliminating any changes over time. Change over time creates a problem when simply comparing the new treatment with historical results (see the story of the Will Rogers phenomenon in Chapter 3).

Some patients may be upset about not being able to choose the new treatment. Randomised studies can only be done if the doctor does not know which treatment is better. When this is the case, any choice of one treatment or the other by a patient will not be based on any known fact but may be just a preference based on other factors such as popular publicity about a new treatment.

Why don't drugs always kill cancer?

Cancers can be resistant to chemotherapy in many ways. Most simply, there are some sites in the body where chemotherapy seems to have more difficulty eradicating the cancer. Such sanctuary sites include the brain and the testicles. We have recognised this because we have seen that, sometimes, when cancers have responded completely everywhere else they have persisted or returned in these sites, suggesting that the tumour didn't respond as well there. This situation can be managed by additional local radiotherapy to these sites in appropriate cases.

There is a genetic mechanism of drug resistance that is quite clever. It confers on the cancer cell resistance to multiple chemotherapy drugs including the anthracyclines, vinca alkaloids, epipodophyllotoxins and taxanes. What they all have in common is that they are natural products. Now, the body didn't know that it would have to deal with cytotoxic drugs. Why would it have this mechanism for resisting them? It is clearly not specific for cytotoxics but forms part of the body's defences against noxious substances in the environment.

The simplified version of the story is that there is a gene called the multidrug resistance gene (MDR) which codes for a protein called p-glycoprotein. Now this protein is in the outer membrane of the cell and acts as a pump. When one of the naturally derived cytotoxics enters the cell, it is pumped out again. This MDR gene and its protein can be switched on to help resist the attack by the cytotoxic drug.

Incidentally, this mechanism can provide another target for new therapies. Can the pump be disabled to overcome the resistance? The pump depends on calcium for its function and initial attempts to overcome resistance were made by combining calcium blockers with the cytotoxic drugs.

Resistance to drugs in other categories depends on how they act. Some drugs, such as methotrexate, rely on an active transport mechanism to get into the cell. Reducing this transport is a simple way of resisting the drug. Another antimetabolite, 5 fluorouracil, needs to be converted to an active form in the cell. Decreasing this conversion will render the drug less effective.

The alkylating agents are made non-toxic by the cell. If that process can be accelerated they will not have time to effect the changes that will lead to the cell's death. Another way for the cell to resist these agents is to repair the damage they cause to the DNA before it is lethal.

As we learn more about what happens between the time that chemotherapy damages the cell's DNA, and the cell's death, there are other pathways that are important in determining the cell's fate. Genes that regulate checkpoints in the cell's reproductive cycle are activated after DNA is damaged. Turning on the p53 gene can determine whether a cell stops to repair itself, enters the reproductive cycle or starts the program that will lead to its death. What genes are turned on, and the balance between the proteins they produce will regulate the program of cell death, or apoptosis, as it is called. Some proteins in this chain of signals can be protective against dying.

Not all the cells in a cancer are the same. With each generation, a group, or clone, of daughter cells may be produced which are more resistant to chemotherapy than their parents. If the cancer is never exposed to chemotherapy, that may not be an advantage. If chemotherapy is given, although much of the tumour will respond, that resistant group will have an advantage over the other cells and survive, frustrating attempts to cure the cancer. This means that if you aim to treat for cure, the chemotherapy should be given as early as possible to minimise the number of times the cancer cells have divided and thus minimise the chance that a resistant clone of cells will arise. It also explains why we give multiple drugs together rather than single agents. Some cells that are resistant to one class of drugs may be killed by another.

The side effects of chemotherapy

The side effects of chemotherapy occur mainly because the drugs attack both the dividing cells in the cancer and those in the remainder of the body. The difference is that the body can often repair itself more efficiently than the cancer. The reason that chemotherapy is frequently given intermittently with three or four weeks between courses is to allow the normal cells to repair themselves between doses.

Most side effects of chemotherapy are reversible and therefore temporary. Some may occur immediately and some years later (see Table 5.2).

We now examine some of these side effects, starting with those that could occur immediately and ending with those that only become apparent after several years.

Extravasation

When a drug is being injected into a vein some leakage, or extravasation, may occur into the tissues around the vein. With many drugs this does not cause a problem. At most, applying ice to the area will limit any discomfort. With other drugs—and the anthracyclines are good examples—what appears of little consequence initially can progress over the following days into a deep ulcer with extensive damage to the skin. This can require a skin graft. With my colleagues, I have shown that the

Table 5.2 Side effects of chemotherapy

In the first 24 hours	Days to weeks	Specific organ drugs	Late effects
Extravasation	Bone marrow suppression	Heart	Second cancers Infertility
Nausea and vomiting	Mouth ulcers	Lungs	Foetal damage
Allergic reaction	Hair loss	Kidney	
		Liver	
		Nervous system	
		Bladder lining	

application of DMSO, an industrial solvent that is available in 44-gallon drums but is also made in purer form for pharmaceutical use, can limit this damage and avoid grafting. Our clinical trial was based on successful animal experiments.

Prevention rather than cure of extravasation should be the aim. Apart from careful technique in needling veins to give chemotherapy, there are now venous access devices, inserted using a quick anaesthetic, which access a large vein in the chest. These devices consist of a reservoir which sits under the skin and a long tube which accesses a vein. They are placed under the skin beneath the collarbone. A needle can be inserted into the reservoir to give chemotherapy by long infusions or for those patients who have small veins in their arms that are difficult to access. Some patients have had a device in place for years but they can be easily removed at the end of several months of chemotherapy.

Allergic reactions

You can be allergic to any drug or substance that you come into contact with and chemotherapy is no exception. Mild allergies would be noticed as flushing or a rash, but severe problems include falls in blood pressure and difficulty in breathing. With a drug such as paclitaxel, the chance of such a reaction is high enough to warrant routinely giving anti-allergy drugs before each dose.

Nausea and vomiting

I have had a longstanding research interest in the control of nausea and vomiting associated with anti-cancer chemotherapy. While not making for great dinner party conversation, it is an area of fascinating complexity where the physical and psychological meet and where great advances have occurred over the past decade.

There are at least three types of vomiting that occur after chemotherapy. The best known is the initial or acute vomiting which occurs within hours of the chemotherapy. Not all cytotoxic drugs make you sick. Some, such as cisplatin, nitrogen mustard and dacarbazine will always cause vomiting. Others, such as cyclophosphamide and doxorubicin, are associated with less severe vomiting, whereas drugs such as vincristine or bleomycin rarely cause vomiting. It is important to realise that there is often a delay of several hours between giving the chemotherapy and becoming sick. Often patients have time to go home before they feel unwell. This vomiting has resolved within 24 hours.

With certain drugs, notably cisplatin, delayed vomiting can occur. This has a different mechanism from acute vomiting. It starts towards the end of the first day and can last for several days.

Finally, there is anticipatory vomiting. This is a learned response. It parallels the classic experiment of Pavlov, in the psychological literature, where he noted that dogs salivated when he brought them food. By ringing a bell prior to the food arriving they eventually salivated when the bell was rung, before the food appeared. Patients feel well, they come to the clinic, receive chemotherapy and become sick. The next time they come in feeling well, they receive chemotherapy which makes them sick, and so on. Eventually, they begin to feel sick just coming to hospital because they associate this with having chemotherapy and becoming sick. In fact, there was a letter to one of the medical journals where an oncologist reported meeting one of his patients in a supermarket, with unfortunate results. The management of this type of vomiting is psychological, trying to decondition patients so that they can continue with their therapy. The best solution is to control the acute vomiting from day one so that the learned response does not occur.

One of the significant advances in the delivery of chemotherapy has been the discovery of a new class of drugs, the serotonin receptor antagonists, which are very effective in the management of acute nausea and vomiting. Chemotherapy causes vomiting by stimulating serotonin receptors in the gut and brain. Again, as a defence against noxious substances, the body seeks to expel the substance by vomiting. These drugs, of which ondansetron was the first example, have few side effects, unlike the older anti-nausea drugs that they replaced. Unfortunately, they are not as effective for delayed emesis so combinations of anti-nausea drugs with steroids are used. More effective treatments are necessary, however.

Some patients are more likely to vomit than others. With cisplatin, women vomit more than men, younger people more than older and those susceptible to motion sickness more than others, while prior exposure to chemotherapy can strongly influence the outcome. Those individuals with a chronically high alcohol intake vomit after chemotherapy less than others!

Suppression of the bone marrow and lowered blood counts

Most of the common chemotherapy drugs cause bone marrow suppression. The bone marrow is where the blood cells are produced. When the drugs are given they kill the cells in the bone marrow that are dividing to replace the older cells that are circulating. They don't kill the mature cells in the bloodstream. The dip in blood counts, mainly of the white blood cells that fight bacterial infections and the platelets that stick together as part of clotting to prevent bleeding, does not occur straight away but ten to fourteen days later. This is when the older cells need to be replaced, but their immediate replacements have been killed by the chemotherapy. Recovery occurs between days 21 and 28 when the next layer of cells in the bone marrow divides and replenishes the blood.

When there is a low white blood cell count, the risk of widespread bacterial infection becomes higher because the body's defences are temporarily down. Any patients who develop a fever over 38^0 Celsius at the time when their white blood count is low will need to be admitted into hospital for intravenous antibiotics, to avoid the risk of overwhelming infection. Cultures of the blood, urine and sputum are performed to see whether the bacteria causing the fever can be identified. Even if they can't, antibiotics covering a broad spectrum of possible organisms have already been commenced and will often start the patient's recovery. Recovery is completed by the return of the white blood cells. Sometimes, the infection can be from organisms found in the mouth or bowel in the patient's body which invade when the defences are down.

How low the blood count goes may depend on the dose of chemotherapy. We could prevent this side effect by decreasing the chemotherapy dose, but this in turn may decrease the effectiveness of the chemotherapy. A significant discovery in this field by Bradley and Metcalf from Australia was the identification of G–CSF (granulocyte colony stimulating factor) which is a growth factor for white cells which fight bacteria. This natural factor can be produced in large quantities and injected in the days following the chemotherapy to stop the white cell counts from falling and thus allow full-dose chemotherapy to be given. When very high doses of chemotherapy are contemplated (which would wipe out the bone marrow), bone marrow or stem cells from the marrow, which circulate in the blood, are collected before the chemotherapy and given back to the patient to restore the bone marrow after the cytotoxic drug treatment.

Low platelet counts increase the risk of bleeding. Very low counts can lead to bleeding without any injury. Patients can be given platelet transfusions, just like red blood cell transfusions, until their platelet counts return to normal. Growth factors that will keep the platelet counts from falling are being developed.

Anaemia, where the red cell counts fall, takes longer to develop and usually occurs slowly over several courses of chemotherapy. Red blood cell transfusions relieve the symptoms of tiredness and breathlessness that develop.

Mouth ulcers

The lining of the mouth, and indeed the whole of the gut, is another area where many of the cells are dividing to replace the cells on the surface. Just as in the bone marrow, the layer of cells that is dividing below the surface is affected by the chemotherapy and about ten days later mouth soreness or ulceration can appear. The degree of ulceration will depend on the dosage of the drugs. The antimetabolites, 5 fluorouracil and methotrexate, are two of the prime candidates for causing this effect. The treatment is to control the symptoms with mouth washes. Secondary infections, particularly with thrush, may make matters worse. Thrush needs specific treatment with antifungal drugs such as nystatin (named because of its development in New York State).

Hair loss

This is perhaps the best known side effect of chemotherapy, but it does not occur with all drugs. Common cytotoxics that cause this are paclitaxel, doxorubicin and cyclophosphamide, whereas chlorambucil and vinblastine rarely cause this problem. Killing dividing cells in the hair follicle causes the hair to become brittle and break off. Not all the hair is lost at once—on the scalp at least 10 per cent of the hairs are in the resting state, while 90 per cent are actively dividing. This means that at least 10 per cent of scalp hairs will not be affected by each dose of treatment and therefore will not fall out two to three weeks following the dose. Almost the opposite occurs on the body where 90 per cent of the hairs may be resting, so early in a course of treatment it appears that only the scalp hairs are lost.

Although preventive measures such as scalp cooling or tourniquets have been tried, they are uncomfortable. They usually only reduce, rather than abolish, hair loss and may, by preventing the blood flow to the scalp during chemotherapy, make it a site for subsequent relapse of the cancer.

The most important message about hair loss with chemotherapy is that it always grows back. It is said to regrow at 0.33 millimetre a day but can be faster in women and slower in the elderly or malnourished. This usually means that three to four months after chemotherapy the hair is long enough for a hairdresser to do something with it. Hair can start regrowing before the end of chemotherapy. The first hair that grows is weak and brittle; it grows back curly but is soon replaced by normally textured hair.

Side effects related to specific organ damage

The side effects discussed so far are common to the majority of cytotoxic drugs. There are some drugs that also have specific side effects by causing damage to organs in the body. For example, each dose of an anthracycline affects the heart muscle so that once a certain cumulative dose is reached, usually after eight or nine doses, the pumping power of the heart can be reduced. Likewise, multiple doses of bleomycin can cause scarring of the lungs. These side effects are well known and serial tests of heart and lung function ensure that the total dose of the drugs can be limited before the damage causes symptoms.

Other effects on the heart include 5 fluorouracil causing spasm of the blood vessels to the heart in a few patients, and cyclophosphamide rarely causing an inflamed heart. The beneficial effects of the drugs usually outweigh these side effects, because they are rare and reversible.

Kidney damage can be caused by cisplatin; it is prevented by giving the drug with fluids, which flushes the drug rapidly through the kidneys. With poor kidney function it may not be possible to administer cisplatin. Methotrexate, which is excreted by the kidneys, may not damage the kidneys but may accumulate, worsening its other side effects. Dose reductions have to occur with these drugs if they are to be given safely in the presence of kidney disease. The bladder can be damaged by cyclophosphamide and ifosfamide. The damage is due to a breakdown product of these drugs and can be prevented by administering the drug with mesna, which inactivates the damaging chemical.

Many drugs are processed by the liver but some—such as the anthracyclines and methotrexate—are toxic to it. The dosage of anthracyclines needs to be reduced if liver function is compromised. Dosages may need to be calculated every time if the liver problems are caused by secondary cancer which is responding to the chemotherapy.

The vinca alkaloids and cisplatin can damage the nerves and cause numbness and tingling in the hands and feet. This takes many months to develop and any improvement occurs very slowly after stopping the drugs. Hearing can also be affected by cisplatin, ranging from ringing in the ears to high frequency hearing loss, which patients notice as difficulty in following a conversation in a crowded noisy room. Effects of cytotoxic drugs on the brain are rarer but can affect balance, muscle strength and brain function.

Late effects of chemotherapy

Some side effects only become apparent months or years after chemotherapy. In males and females sterility can occur. This most commonly happens with alkylating agents but is by no means an all-or-nothing phenomenon. There are many reports of normal healthy children being born after one parent has received prior chemotherapy. We usually advise a gap of two years after chemotherapy. This allows repair of damage but also helps determine the likely outcome of the treatment, which may help us decide whether the parent is likely to survive to raise the child. Sperm can be collected prior to chemotherapy and stored. Often, however, the sperm count is found to be low before the chemotherapy, as an indirect result of having the cancer.

We try hard to avoid giving chemotherapy during pregnancy because of the potential damage to the foetus. Certainly, it should not be given in the first trimester but occasionally the less damaging drugs may be given later in the pregnancy if the mother's life is at risk.

Just as with radiotherapy, another long-term risk of chemotherapy is the development of a second cancer. The average time after chemotherapy is about four years, which means that this group of patients have usually been cured of their original cancer. The most common second malignancy is leukaemia, but lymphomas and solid cancers can occur. Although we must not compromise the chance of curing the original tumour by reducing the therapy, we do know that the use of alkylating agents, prolonged treatments and combining chemotherapy with radiotherapy increases the risk of developing second cancers. We try to develop new treatments that avoid these scenarios.

When do we use chemotherapy?

When you read through a list of the possible side effects you may well wonder whether the cure is worse than the disease. The decision to start chemotherapy is a balance between the likely risks and benefits. Most of the side effects of chemotherapy are temporary, whereas there could be a significant long-term benefit if the symptoms caused by cancer are controlled. There are several situations where chemotherapy is used.

Chemotherapy can be used as adjuvant, or additional, treatment following definitive local treatment, be that surgery or radiotherapy. Adjuvant chemotherapy is aimed at treating microscopic disease that may have escaped prior to the local treatment and be responsible for the disease returning later. Occasionally, the chemotherapy can be given before the local treatment to shrink the disease and increase the chances of cure.

Most chemotherapy is given for widespread or metastatic disease. Rarely in this setting is it curative, but important exceptions include testicular cancer, lymphomas and childhood tumours (see Table 5.3).

Table 5.3 Efficacy of chemotherapy

Potentially curative	Can achieve control	Relatively restricted
Childhood leukaemia	Breast cancer	Kidney cancer
Childhood Wilm's tumour	Small cell lung cancer	Melanoma
Childhood sarcomas	Bladder cancer	Bowel cancer
Choriocarcinoma	Low grade lymphoma	Liver cancer
Hodgkin's lymphoma	Myeloma	Prostate cancer
Non-Hodgkin's lymphoma	Chronic leukaemia	Non-small cell lung cancer
Testicular cancer	Head and neck cancer	
	Sarcoma	

Where cure is the aim, chemotherapy must be started as soon as practicable to lessen the chance that resistance will develop. The main aim of most chemotherapy, then, is to shrink the disease and control it for as long as possible. When making a decision about when to use chemotherapy, we must balance the fact that it will be more effective if we treat earlier when the cancer is smaller with the reality that patients who are having no symptoms from a cancer will be made to feel temporarily worse if they have side effects from chemotherapy. Even those with some symptoms from the cancer may have them easily relieved with simple medication, although this will not attack the cause of the symptom. Patients given all the necessary information will make their decisions about therapy based on their own priorities and philosophy of life.

Regional chemotherapy

We have focused mainly on chemotherapy designed to circulate throughout the body. There are some special circumstances where it can be given into just one region of the body. For example, if multiple deposits of melanoma are confined to a limb, the limb can be isolated by putting a tube into the artery supplying it and another in the vein draining it. High-dose chemotherapy can then be injected into the artery and drained out by the vein without circulating around the body. The techniques are being refined and the extent of the advantage to this approach, as compared with systemic chemotherapy, is difficult to determine.

The liver provides us with another opportunity for injecting high doses of drugs directly into its artery without doing too much damage to the normal cells, or the rest of the body. Here, the normal cells are protected by the fact that they have an alternate blood supply from the portal vein which drains from the bowels. The drugs used are cleared by the liver as they pass through it, with only some getting out into the rest of the circulation. This intrahepatic chemotherapy is only useful if you are sure that all the cancer you want to control is confined to the liver.

The other situation for regional chemotherapy is when the disease is present in a confined cavity in the body. Drugs can be introduced into the abdominal cavity, for example. Cancer affecting the lining of the brain and spinal cord, the meninges, can be treated by injecting a drug into the fluid that surrounds those structures. Both these situations allow the local tissues to be exposed to high concentrations of a drug without damaging the rest of the body.

Combined treatments

We mentioned that chemotherapy can be given before or after radiotherapy. It can also be an advantage to give it at the same time as radiotherapy. This can increase the side effects but also the benefits. The drugs to be used in this situation must be carefully selected. We have already seen that cisplatin can sensitise the cancer to the effects of the radiotherapy, which can be a great advantage. Care must be taken with other drugs. Anthracyclines can significantly increase the local burning effect of radiotherapy. Even if given after radiotherapy, the anthra-cyclines can make the local irradiated area red again in a recall of the previous side effects.

Is more better?

There are two ways of increasing the intensity of chemotherapy. One is to give a larger dose. The other is to give the chemotherapy over a longer time. The problem with giving a larger dose are the side effects, which limit the dose that can be given. Not all drugs are suitable for high-dose treatment. Any drug that works only in a particular part of the cell cycle can kill only the cells that are at that step; therefore, increasing the dose does not help. Drugs that disrupt DNA in any phase of the cell cycle, such as the alkylating agents, are ideal candidates. The next consideration is what side effects the drug will have.

If the main side effect of a drug is bone marrow suppression, then the use of the patient's own bone marrow or peripheral blood stem cells for transplant with growth factor support allows escalation of the dose. Alkylating agents fit this description. There is now a series of trials in lymphomas and solid cancers where high-dose drug combinations are given with rescue of the marrow. The bone marrow is harvested before the procedure; or the stem cells are collected by taking blood from the patient, separating the stem cells from the other blood cells and returning the remainder to the patient. The number of stem cells available for collection can be increased by giving a dose of chemotherapy or growth factors to stimulate their production before the collection is due. In leukaemias, where the treatment involves destroying the marrow which contains the leukaemic cell, donated marrow is used. This is discussed further in Chapter 7.

The development of small portable infusion pumps, which can be worn clipped to a patient's belt and which contain a small bag of chemotherapy, has allowed prolonged infusions of chemotherapy drugs to be developed. It doesn't matter if the drug is specific for a particular event in the cell's reproductive cycle, because the drug is infused continuously and the cancer cells will be exposed as they enter the cycle.

The drug, 5 fluorouracil, is commonly used in this way and can be delivered for months at a time. It can be more effective than when given as a single dose and the side effects are fewer, since the dose at any one time is low; for any side effect that is bothersome the pump can be switched off. It is interesting that when delivered in this way the side effects are different from those seen with short doses. With 5 fluorouracil, mouth ulcers and diarrhoea become dose-limiting; pain, redness and peeling of the hands and feet are seen only with this prolonged schedule.

HORMONE THERAPY

Hormones are chemical messengers. Some organs are under the influence of hormones released from other areas of the body. For example, an area in the brain called the hypothalamus can stimulate the pituitary gland beneath the brain to release hormones which act in turn on the ovary or testicle to produce the female hormones, oestrogens, or the male hormones, androgens. Organs that are sensitive to these sex hormones include breast tissue, the endometrium (i.e. the lining of the uterus) and the prostate gland. The cancers that are most widely treated with hormones arise in these tissues. It is estimated that 15 per cent of all cancers respond to hormones. The first recorded cases of cancers being responsive to hormones were in three patients whose breast cancer was reported by George Beatson from Glasgow in 1896 to have responded to removal of the ovaries.

Hormone treatment is designed to interfere with the normal hormone-stimulated growth of the cancers and results in the cancer dying. Let us take breast cancer as an example. Breast cancers respond to oestrogens. Tamoxifen is a drug that competes with oestrogen for the oestrogen receptor (ER) in the cells. Stimulation of this receptor usually activates oestrogen-sensitive genes in the nucleus of the cell, but when this process is blocked the cell can die. Some of the effects of oestrogen can occur when tamoxifen binds to the receptor, so that we see some oestrogen effects on the blood fats and the density of the bones, but mainly we see the cancer die because the tamoxifen has blocked the ability of oestrogen to stimulate the cancer. Some cells will be resistant to tamoxifen—not all cells express oestrogen receptors, or there may be alterations in the pathways stimulated via the ER.

Tamoxifen is a tablet that is used in both the adjuvant setting after local surgery or radiotherapy, and to control advanced disease, in those breast cancers which are found to have oestrogen receptors. In the adjuvant setting it should be used for at least five years. It has few side effects but can cause vaginal discharge or dryness. There has been concern that prolonged use may increase the occurrence of cancers of the endometrium. Occasionally, when first given, tamoxifen can cause a flare-up of bone pain, but this settles spontaneously and can precede a response. Responses can take weeks to see and so hormone treatments are not chosen if vital organs are threatened and a rapid response is required.

Progestogens such as medroxyprogesterone acetate (MPA) can be used as a second-choice hormone for breast cancer, after tamoxifen. They have a variety of actions affecting oestrogen synthesis and breakdown and can kill the cancer cells. A side effect of MPA is weight gain. This has been utilised to treat weight loss in cancers that do not respond to hormones.

The ovaries are not the only site of production of oestrogenic hormones. The adrenal gland is also responsible for some production. A series of hormones called aromatase inhibitors can block the adrenal production of oestrogen in women after the menopause and prevent the growth of sensitive breast cancers. The first of these, aminoglutethimide, can have uncomfortable side effects including sickness, low blood pressure and rash. Because of the suppression of the adrenal gland, the steroid, hydrocortisone, has to be taken with the aminoglutethimide. This is not necessary with the newer drugs in this class.

The story with prostate cancer is similar. The gold standard method of preventing the stimulation of the prostate by male androgens was to remove the testicles. Now stimulation of the prostate can be prevented with hormone injections or tablets that disrupt the production pathways of the male hormone. Injections of the gonadotrophin-releasing hormones (which mimic those hormones from the hypothalamus that stimulate the pituitary gland) can deplete the stores in the pituitary and prevent the stimulation of the testicles to produce the androgens.

Initially, there can be a surge of androgens causing a flare-up of the cancer symptoms, but this can be treated with an anti-androgen such as flutamide which blocks androgen receptors.

A large randomised trial has found that there is no benefit to the use of an anti-androgen in addition to surgery to remove the testicles. This finding showed the benefit of such trials, since it had been common practice to do the surgery and commence an anti-androgen. Current trials are investigating a whole range of hormones that have greater efficacy and less toxicity than those currently in use.

TREATMENT OF CANCER WITH 'NATURAL' BIOLOGICAL AGENTS

Biological therapy for cancer attempts either to make use of the body's defence mechanisms to kill cancer cells or to use substances produced by cells that are part of the body's immune system. Although these are the products of nature it may be misleading to call the treatments 'natural'. Some of the substances can be produced outside the body and given back to the patient at many times the concentration in which they would normally be found. This means they can have side effects just like many manufactured drugs. It is rather like claiming that huge doses of vitamins are natural because smaller doses are a non-toxic part of a normal diet.

The immune system

The immune system is a complex defence system designed to recognise anything that is foreign to the normal body. The trouble with tumours is that they often don't produce much of an immune response because they are too like the normal body. Immune cells are mainly types of white blood cells (e.g. lymphocytes) which circulate through the blood, lymph channels and tissues. They produce antibodies which are proteins that can specifically recognise target proteins called antigens on the cells that the body needs to be immunised against. Some of the immune cells also produce proteins called cytokines or inter-leukins, which means 'between white cells', and that describes exactly what they do. Interleukins are produced in tiny amounts but carry messages between cells that are part of the immune system and regulate the complex events that are part of the body's defence system.

There are many ways in which the killing of foreign cells can occur. An immune cell can interact with the antigens on a foreign cell and kill it. If antibodies bind to a foreign cell it can help scavenger cells recognise it as foreign and destroy it. Lymphocytes can be killer cells if they are exposed to a particular interleukin, IL–2, and interleukins themselves can kill some cells.

Immunotherapy

It is an attractive idea to use the body's own defence mechanisms to kill a cancer. Some cancers have been known to disappear without treatment, causing speculation that the immune system played a role. Serial observations of patients with multiple melanoma deposits or secondary deposits from kidney cancer, for example, have occasionally revealed these spontaneous shrinkages. Early attempts to stimulate the body's immune system were based on William Coley's observation early in the twentieth century that tumours would shrink in patients who developed an infection. The idea was that if you could rev up the immune system against an infective agent (e.g. bacillus Calmette-Guerin, BCG, used to stimulate the immune system against TB) it would also act against cancer. Despite early reports of success, when tested in randomised clinical trials these approaches did not work. Non-specific stimulation of the immune system was not able to kill cancer, and I suspect the same is true for a number of unproven therapies and diets that have as their rationale stimulation of the immune system. The only exception seems to be in the treatment of local cancers. Injecting BCG under melanomas or instilling it into a bladder to kill superficial tumours of the bladder lining has proved successful.

Tumour vaccines

Tumour vaccines are an attempt to target the tumour more specifically. It is possible to immunise mice using cancer cells or parts of cells. This may prevent the growth of a new cancer but does not kill an already established cancer. With increasing knowledge of how the immune system responds, there has been a new interest in tumour vaccines. Tumour cells don't stimulate much of an immune response themselves but this can be improved. Tumour cells injected with certain interleukins or growth factors produce a greater immune response from the body. Genes can be introduced or altered in cancer cells to make the cells more able to stimulate the body's immune system against the cancer.

It is known that a certain type of lymphocyte called a T-lymphocyte is specific for cancer target antigens and can be stimulated to kill cancers by injecting tumour cells with IL–2. Vaccines are being developed specifically to obtain an immune response that utilises these cells.

Tumour antigens can be common to cancers from different patients. This means that instead of having to produce a vaccine for each patient from pieces of their own cancers, which is very labour-intensive, vaccines could be made from cancer cells that are kept alive in the laboratory for the purpose. There are many proteins in the cells that are tumour-specific and are recognised by T-cells and these proteins can become very specific targets for vaccines.

Different approaches to obtaining the antigens that are used to produce the vaccine will each have advantages and disadvantages, which illustrates the difficulty of developing tumour vaccines. If you decide to prepare a vaccine from a biopsy of a patient's tumour, you may find you have unique antigens for that patient that would not form part of a vaccine from a related tumour. You have the disadvantage, though, that you have sampled only one part of the tumour, which may be different in other parts, and a cancer straight from a patient may not be capable of eliciting a strong immune response. If you use a vaccine made from a number of cell lines kept in the laboratory you can cover some of the variability in tumours and manipulate the cancer cells to make them more likely to stimulate an immune response. A major disadvantage is that there may be a strong response against the foreign cells which prevent a response against the shared tumour antigens. If you try the third option and manufacture a vaccine against a limited number of tumour-specific proteins, the tumour may be more easily able to change itself and avoid recognition by the immune system.

Theoretically, producing a tumour-specific vaccine should be an ideal way to kill a cancer. However, with great variability within a cancer, the weak immune response to a cancer, and the ability of a cancer cell to change so that it can't be recognised by the immune system, or to produce local immune suppressants to prevent an immune response, the clinical benefit is not assured. Patients with cancer may already have poor immune systems, either because of the cancer or because of previous therapy. Despite all this, there have been some encouraging results in trials of vaccines. Many of the initial trials focused on melanoma, but vaccines are now being tested in many other cancers, both to prevent recurrence and to shrink established cancers.

Interferons

Interferons are proteins initially found to be produced by cells in response to a viral infection. They prevent the patient from being infected with a second virus. They have a number of effects on the immune system and the growth of tumours and can kill cancer cells directly. They are active against some lymphomas and chronic leukaemias and have limited activity against selected solid cancers. Some studies have reported improved survival in patients who received interferon to prevent melanomas returning.

Monoclonal antibodies

It is possible, using a clever, yet simple, technique to produce antibodies that target specific antigens on cancers. These are called monoclonal antibodies because they are all of the one type and specific for an antigen on the surface of the cancer cell. They should not bind to other antigens on other cells. These antibodies have great potential. If they have the ability to kill cancer cells they can be used directly to do that. If not, they can be linked to a drug or a poison or a source of radioactivity and be used to target the lethal agent to the tumour. They can also be used in similar fashion for the diagnosis of cancers by tagging them with an isotope and then scanning the patient. It is hoped they could detect small deposits of cancer that would otherwise be missed by conventional scanning.

Problems can occur if the antibody has been produced in another species, such as a mouse, since the human body could then produce antibodies against the monoclonal antibody. Often, not much of the injected antibody reaches the tumour and what does may have trouble penetrating into the middle of large cancers. Sometimes, they can be mopped up by antigens before they get to the tumour. There are potential problems if the antigen they target can also be found on normal cells.

Interleukin 2

Interleukin 2 (IL–2) is one of the cytokines produced by lymphocytes that can regulate the immune response. It can stimulate lymphocytes so they are able to kill cancers. It has no direct killing effect on cancers but acts through the immune system. It seems to stimulate the production of other cytokines that are important in the immune system. In the clinic IL–2 was used primarily with the adoptive transfer of immune cells. That is, the patient's lymphocytes were exposed to IL–2 which turned them into killer cells. When given back to the patient, responses were seen particularly in melanoma and kidney cancer.

Tumour-infiltrating lymphocytes

Tumour-infiltrating lymphocytes (TILs) are lymphocytes that are seen to home in on cancers. They can be isolated from the cancer and then injected back into a patient. Because they home in on tumours, attempts are being made to alter them genetically to make them more poisonous to the cancer they target.

Gene therapy

Gene therapy is a treatment that involves inserting a functioning gene into a cell. Often this has to be done outside the body and the cells replaced in the body. First, the gene has to be inserted into a cell. There are many techniques, but one borrowed from nature is to use a virus to insert the gene—viruses multiply by inserting the genetic code for copying themselves into a cell and using the cell's machinery to divide. Once the gene is in the cell, it is hoped that the product it codes for is produced by the cell.

The potential of this technology is large. Just as one example, tumour-infiltrating lymphocytes could have their genetic characteristics changed to enhance their sensitivity to other growth factors so that more can be produced. Tumours could be targeted directly by inserting a gene that would produce a product that caused a cancer cell to die. A cancer that lost a tumour suppressor gene could have it replaced. The scenarios are endless and much research is being performed into this new treatment modality.

NEW TARGETS FOR TREATMENT

The growth of a cancer can be disrupted at many points. Many of our cytotoxic drugs disrupt DNA. There are techniques for targeting very specifically the piece of genetic material being disrupted. If a complementary strand of genetic material is made for a length of messenger RNA and binds to it, there is no way that the message can be used to produce the product. The strand is called an antisense length of genetic material because it blocks the 'sense' message of the RNA. Clinical trials have already been performed with such antisense drugs.

A further innovative strategy for conquering a cancer focuses on curbing the growth and the ability of a cancer to spread. We alluded earlier to drugs that prevent the new blood vessels forming that the tumour needs in order to grow and spread. These so-called anti-angiogenesis factors have been shown in clinical trials to retard cancer growth, with very few side effects.

SUMMARY

Cancer treatments include those that will achieve local control of a cancer and cure of localised disease and those that can act throughout the body. Surgery and radiotherapy were discussed as the local treatments. Systemic treatments include chemo-therapy, hormone therapy and biological therapies. The treatment modalities can be combined in sequence or given together. The newer approaches to conquering cancer explore specific immune therapies and gene therapies. They also search for new targets to disrupt cancer growth, such as preventing formation of the new blood vessels required by the cancer.

6

The spectrum of cancers

Variety's the very spice of life, that gives it all its flavour.

—*William Cowper*

What are the most common types of cancer? Which cancers most often result in death? Cancer is a family of illnesses with common features but great diversity. We have spoken of there being over 100 different types, some common, some rare. We can study individual cancers but for an overall grasp of how cancer behaves it is important to have an overview of the broad spectrum of cancers. Epidemiology is the name given to the study of the overall population distribution of cancer and what determines when and where the disease will occur.

EPIDEMIOLOGY

We first met epidemiology when we discussed the causes of cancer. The information collected by epidemiologists describes the occurrence of cancer and how that changes over time. Theories of why the changes have occurred are then tested by analysing the information to try to identify the risk factors for developing cancer. Finally, you can use the information

137

collected from the whole population to assess whether prevention, screening or treatment programs are impacting on the incidence of a cancer or the deaths from it.

CANCER REGISTRIES

Information about the occurrence of cancer in the whole population is collected by cancer registries. To be useful, cancer registries must collect data on all the cancers in the area they serve. The idea is not new, originating from the turn of the century, but registration of cancers in whole populations started in the 1940s. Now registries exist all around the world. Each is established to service a defined geographical area, such as a small country or a state. Population-based cancer registries are quite different from hospital-based registries. Hospitals keep data on their own patients without necessarily knowing how that data relates to the whole population. The information collected is very useful for administration when deciding what resources need to be put into cancer care. It can also be used to identify cases so that outcomes of care can be measured. A population-based registry has data that may be more useful for community health planning, including prevention strategies.

How does a registry identify all the cases? Governments could make it mandatory to report cancer, just as some infectious diseases must be reported, or the reporting could be voluntary. Busy doctors can be very slow filling in forms. The case capture rate is often more complete by downloading data from pathology services at the time the cancer is initially diagnosed.

In this computer age there is a deal of paranoia about government data collections and issues of privacy and confidentiality. It has been argued that such collections may compromise individual rights for the benefit of the community. I regard this as nonsense. First, we all live in the community and benefit from the cancer control initiatives that stem from cancer registry-based information. More important, however, is the

138

information that the cancer registry gives individuals about the outcomes of cancer management in the community in which they live. They can compare this with other states or countries and judge whether their local health care system is up to scratch.

A population-based cancer registry is not interested in individual cases but in the cancer figures of the population as a whole group. It doesn't collect detailed information but is more intent on collecting basic information completely. A typical registry will collect information about the person such as name, sex, race and date of birth and information about the cancer such as date of diagnosis, and type and site of the cancer. The date of death of the person is often most simply obtained through a register of births, deaths and marriages which then allows survival times to be calculated. At the population level there is usually no information about treatment. The initial treatment and outcome of that treatment is the information that a hospital registry would collect. Ideally, the two collections could be linked to create a more comprehensive database.

CANCER INCIDENCE AND MORTALITY

The incidence of cancer refers to the rate at which new cases of cancer are diagnosed over a period of time. This is usually recorded as a rate for every 100 000 of the population. The mortality is the number of deaths from cancer over a particular time, again expressed as a number for every 100 000 of population. These rates can be compared between registries, although they should be corrected for age first to ensure that the populations being compared are alike.

It is estimated that around the world seven million new cases of cancer will be diagnosed each year. In the Western world more than half the cancers are from four sites: lung, large bowel, prostate and breast. If I take some figures from my home state South Australian registry as an example, prostate cancer was the leading male cancer accounting for 25 per cent of the male cancers. Large bowel cancer represented 15 per cent of male cancers followed by lung and then melanoma, which has a high incidence in Australia. If you look at the mortality figures for males, lung cancer causes the most deaths followed by prostate and large bowel cancer. By comparison, breast cancer has the highest incidence in females, representing 27 per cent of cancers in women, followed by large bowel, melanoma and lung. Breast cancer is still the major cause of death in women, ahead of lung cancer and bowel cancer.

The overall figures for all cancer sites show that 52 per cent of patients diagnosed with cancer will be alive five years later, which is very similar to United States figures. There is a gender difference with the figures showing 57 per cent for females and 46 per cent for males. People under 55 years also have a higher survival than those over 75 years, the five-year survival rates being 68 per cent and 41 per cent respectively. Some pessimists who believe that cancer is a death sentence will be surprised at these figures. They indicate that most cancers should be con-sidered as chronic rather than acute diseases. Even if we can't cure as many cancers as we would wish to, we may still control them for a long time.

Some patients misinterpret the five-year mark as being significant for their cancer. It is merely a convention to choose the five-year mark to compare one country's figures with another. Mind you, the rate of drop-off between five and ten or fifteen years is small, with 47 per cent of the population quoted above surviving at both time points.

Collecting information over many years allows examination of the trends in both the incidence and mortality of cancer. The South Australian figures, for example, indicate that survival has improved. The age-adjusted five-year survival for the years 1977 to 1985 was 47 per cent, compared with 53 per cent for 1986 to 1994.

Trends in the United States are reflected in other Western countries. In females the lung cancer incidence and mortality have more than doubled in the last two decades. It is thought that this is due to the increasing number of women who have taken up smoking in the years following the Second World

War. A rise in lymphomas was seen as AIDS became more widespread, since lymphomas and Kaposi's sarcomas are both found in association with this disease that suppresses the immune system. A large increase in the incidence of prostate cancer has been recorded. This could be explained by the increased utilisation of screening tests which are now detecting the very early disease before symptoms develop. The rising incidence of breast cancer may be partly explained by earlier detection, but changes in practices in the use of contraceptives and breast feeding may be part of a more complex story.

On the positive side, the incidence and mortality from cancer of the cervix has declined. This is almost certainly related to early detection through the Pap smear program and successful treatment of early disease. The decreasing incidence and mortality from stomach cancer is more difficult to explain. Some of the reasons suggested have included changes in dietary and socioeconomic factors as well as populations migrating away from areas of high incidence to countries with a lower incidence of the disease. A lower death rate is being noted for testicular cancer and Hodgkin's lymphoma. Given that these two diseases have a high chance of responding to chemotherapy, improved treatment is the most likely factor to explain the improvement in death rate. Our previous discussion about the need to do randomised trials to prove that a treatment, and not other factors, causes the improved result shows that the statistics collected by an epidemiologist cannot be used for anything more than suggesting reasons for change. It is possible to test theories on a population basis.

ANALYSING EPIDEMIOLOGICAL DATA

When analysing the data collected by epidemiologists, statistical associations can be found between a cancer and a possible risk factor. This does not mean that the factor is a cause of the cancer. It may, for example, simply be related to another factor that is the cause. In a hypothetical case, say that you found an association between stress and lung cancer. It would not be possible to say that stress is a cause of lung cancer. It may be that people who are stressed smoke more than those who are not. The actual causative factor is smoking, and stress is just related.

Another example could be the observation that people who eat a Western diet that has a high fat content with little fibre are more prone to bowel cancer than inhabitants of developing countries who rely more on high-fibre fruit and vegetable diets. The diet may play a key role but you can't make that assumption simply on an observed difference between the incidences of bowel cancer. There may be other differences. For example, if the figures are not corrected for age it may be that more people die young with infectious diseases in developing countries and don't reach the older age group where bowel cancer is the most common.

As it happened, the theory of the influence of diet on bowel cancer was verified in another way. Studies of Japanese migrants going to the United States showed that when they changed their diets from rice to burgers and fries they adopted the higher bowel cancer risk within one generation. This suggested that an environmental factor was at play and diet was the prime suspect. If the change in environment helps trigger the development of cancer by affecting children when they are growing, then it takes at least one generation in the new country before there is a change in the incidence of cancer in the immigrant population.

Case-controlled and cohort studies

To obtain evidence of an association between a potential risk factor and the development of cancer from epidemiological data, we can't easily use randomised clinical trials. Unlike cancer treatments, where the outcomes of death or recurrence are frequent, in a healthy population the incidence of a specific cancer is low so that a study would have to be very large and would require a long time to follow up all the cases. Instead, epidemiologists rely on cohort and case-controlled studies. They try to find out the relative risk of developing cancer, or how many times greater the risk of cancer is if you are exposed to a potentially causative agent compared with a situation in which you are not exposed.

Cohort studies, which follow people over many years, identify groups of individuals from a population who are either exposed or not exposed to a particular factor. These individuals are then followed until sufficient cancers have occurred to allow the numbers in the exposed group to be compared with the numbers in the unexposed group. The relative risk can be calculated from these two groups. These studies may be set up in advance to study the two groups, or done by looking back at records of exposure and disease recurrence. Sometimes, just the background population incidence and mortality rates are used as points of comparison with the exposed group.

Case studies start from people who have cancer and a matched group who do not and then extract information about prior exposure to the agent in question (e.g. passive smoking). The proportion of cases who have had the exposure are compared with those who have not. The major challenge of a case-controlled study is to select the controls from a similar population who will have had the same chance of exposure to the agent being investigated. If the cancer group has been selected from a hospital population then the control group could be other patients matched with the cancer patients in every characteristic except for having cancer. If the cancer group had come from the general population then the controls could be found by randomly sampling the general population to find individuals who match the cancer patients.

There are pros and cons for each approach. Cohort studies trace the development over time after exposure but take a long time to do. Case-control studies are more prone to bias in recalling exposure, since patients with cancer may remember exposures in a way that those without would not. These studies have the advantage of generally being based on larger numbers than cohort studies. Evidence for the cause of a cancer needs to be seen in not just one but several epidemiological studies that show the same thing. It is important to remember, too, that these studies apply to whole populations and do not dictate the outcomes for individual cases.

SPECIFIC CANCERS

To illustrate the variability of cancers and the application of epidemiological studies, we now look at some of the common cancers in men and women.

Prostate cancer

This cancer shows great variation geographically. It is the most common cancer in the United States, northern Europe and Australia but is rare in Asia and Africa. In America the incidence and mortality are nearly twice as high in blacks as in whites. Japanese migrants to California show an increase in the incidence of prostate cancer but not to the level of the Americans. The variability is seen in clinically detectable prostate cancer; the finding of 'silent' prostate cancer either by screening or at post-mortem examination is less variable. The only risk factors supported by strong data are age, race and family history.

Other factors that have been suggested as causative include higher sex hormone levels and sexual activity, but this is unproven. Dietary fat has been implicated but this can impact on male hormone levels. There is no convincing evidence that smoking and prostate cancer are linked. It is clear that this is a cancer where much more study of its behaviour and causation is required.

Bladder cancer

Although not one of the common cancers (it is the eighth commonest in males), I will discuss bladder cancer while we are in its vicinity. Unlike prostate cancer, black Americans have half the incidence of white Americans. The bladder is exposed to the breakdown products of many chemicals taken into the body and these exposures could cause cancer. Epidemiological studies have suggested occupational exposure to substances such as dyes may cause bladder cancer, while there is mixed evidence on the relationship with coffee drinking. There is some evidence that a fresh fruit and vegetable diet may be protective. We have already discussed exposure to the cytotoxic drug cyclophosphamide as being a causative factor. A major risk factor identified from epidemiological studies is cigarette smoking. The risk is associated with the 'dose' of cigarettes and parallels the geographic areas of high incidence. Epidemiological studies can, therefore, not only indicate causes but provide the information upon which prevention strategies can be based.

I want to illustrate the point that even cancers of the same organ can't just be considered indiscriminately. Exposure to the parasite Schistosoma haemotobium is a major cause of bladder cancer in Africa and the Middle East. Whereas most bladder cancer comes from the transitional cells that line the bladder, association with the parasite gives rise to a completely different type of bladder cancer, made of squamous cells, which behaves in quite a different way; we would not expect it to be associated with the same risk factors.

Cancer of the cervix

This is the second most important cause of cancer in women across the world. The highest rates are in South America, Africa and South-East Asia, with low rates in Israel; unlike other cancers we have discussed, no country has very low rates. The incidence and mortality have decreased as early changes in the cervix detected by the smear test are adequately treated (see Chapter 4).

The risk factors identified from epidemiological studies parallel those for a sexually transmitted disease. Early age of first intercourse, multiple sexual partners, multiple pregnancies, long-term contraceptive use, lower socioeconomic status and

145

smoking are all risk factors. These have been increasingly strongly linked to infection with the human papilloma virus.

Good diet with an emphasis on fruit and vegetables may be protective, either because of its components or because a good diet is associated with other aspects of a healthy lifestyle.

Breast cancer

Breast cancer has the highest incidence of cancers in women in many Western nations, although its incidence is lower in South-east Asia but is now being overtaken by lung cancer as the greatest cause of death in women. Many of the risk factors determined by large epidemiological studies seem to be related to the exposure of the breast to female hormones. The risk of breast cancer becomes greater as the onset of menstrual cycles becomes earlier and menopause later, and not having been pregnant, while an early first full-term pregnancy is protective. Again I remind you that this applies to populations and is not meant to advocate an individual woman having an early pregnancy to protect herself from breast cancer! The oral contraceptive pill has not been causative of breast cancer in most epidemiological studies. Prolonged hormone replacement therapy in postmenopausal women is associated with a slightly increased risk of breast cancer.

Breast cancer again illustrates the lack of clarity in the information available from population-based epidemiological studies. Obesity is a risk factor in women after menopause but it may be the inverse in premenopausal women. Eating a diet rich in fat cannot be demonstrated as a lifelong risk factor. Whether exposure at specific times, such as adolescence, is important has not been determined. Exercise may, however, be beneficial in reducing the risk of breast cancer. Alcohol consumption has proved in many studies to increase the risk of developing breast cancer.

Other risk factors that have emerged from population studies include a strong family history (see Chapter 2). Previous benign changes in the breast have also been found to predispose to breast cancer, and radiation exposure is a factor where the risk increases as time passes. It will take prolonged observation of many groups of patients to resolve the outstanding issues related to hormone and dietary exposure.

Lung cancer

Lung cancer has the highest incidence of any cancer worldwide and has been a leading cause of cancer death in males. The death rate in women is increasing rapidly. Epidemiological studies over the last 50 years have found that smoking tobacco is the major risk factor. Extensive campaigns to warn of the risk of smoking and the benefits of quitting seem to be working in adult males but not as well in teenagers, particularly teenage girls. Passive smoking, by being in a confined space filled with cigarette smoke, is also a risk factor which is driving regulations to ban smoking in enclosed public places or transport vehicles.

Smoking cigarettes increases the risk if the smoker is also exposed to other possible causative agents. Heading the list is radiation, either from radon gas or accidental exposure to nuclear fallout.

A diet of fruit and vegetables may be of benefit in reducing the risk of cancer in smokers. Of interest is the suggestion that some individuals may have a genetic reason for being at less risk of smoking-related cancer, depending on the ease with which they can break down the cancer-causing chemicals in cigarette smoke.

Large bowel cancer

Large bowel cancer is the third most common cancer in the world. There is a similar incidence in men and women. The disease is frequent in the United States and northern Europe, but low in Africa. This is an interesting disease to illustrate the use and limitations of epidemiology. The lower bowel, or rectum, behaves somewhat differently from the upper bowel but is often included with it in population studies.

147

We saw earlier that there can be inherited factors, but the study of people who have migrated to areas of different incidence indicates that environmental factors are very important. After migrating to Israel, Jewish men born in America have a higher incidence of bowel cancer than those born in Africa. The children of Japanese migrants in America have an incidence of bowel cancer approaching that of the children of American parents.

The major risk factors are dietary and each can be plausibly explained, but it is difficult to dissect out details. Let us take the association with fat intake. There is also an association with increased energy intake from overeating, or alcohol, although not necessarily with obesity. Also, people who exercise more have a lower incidence of bowel cancer. As it happens, fat intake is a risk factor independent of total energy. However, it is not all fats that are important, but specifically animal fats. It can be recommended, then, that high-fat red meats be replaced with fish or chicken. Red meats, though, may not be a risk factor just because of their fat content; cooked red meats may have cancer-causing chemicals in them in their own right.

It is easy to suggest a mechanism for a diet high in animal fat causing bowel cancer. Fat turns on bile acids which alter bacteria in the gut and increase the concentration of chemicals that can promote cancer. In a final twist of irony, however, low blood cholesterol has been reported as a risk factor for bowel cancer. It is unlikely to be a cause but just an association that has been found in population-based studies.

It has been suggested that increased dietary fibre can protect against bowel cancer—based on differences in bowel cancer risk in countries with different fibre intakes. Of course, this is not the only difference between these populations as discussed earlier in this chapter. A plausible explanation can be offered for fibre protecting against bowel cancer. Increased fibre causes the bowel motions to be more bulky, which enables them to be pushed through the bowel more quickly, reducing the time that any cancer-causing chemicals remain in contact with the bowel. Fibre comes from many sources and, much to the chagrin of breakfast cereal manufacturers, it is the fibre from fruits and vegetables that seems to be the favoured foodstuff.

Other vitamins and trace elements, including vitamin E, selenium and beta carotene, have been suggested as protective. This is not to say that these substances would be useful in treating established cancer. However, it is exciting that epidemiological studies can offer suggestions for the prevention of cancer—we return to this later.

Stomach cancer

I want to discuss stomach cancer because it is the second most frequent form of cancer in the world. It has a very high incidence in Japan but, fortunately, the incidence has been decreasing steadily all over the world over the past four or five decades. This is another cancer where migrating from a high-incidence area to a low-incidence area changes the risk in the migrating people.

The dietary habits of those in high-risk countries include the ingestion of starchy foods and foods preserved by salting or smoking. In more affluent areas, a diet of fruit and vegetables seems protective. The theory is that some preserving methods, such as salting, increase the nitrosamine content of the food which stays in prolonged contact with the gastric mucosa. Some of the vitamins in fresh fruit and vegetables can inhibit these nitroso compounds. A further possible explanation of the decrease in the incidence of the disease could be the introduction of better ways of preserving food as refrigeration becomes widespread.

Another factor associated with stomach cancer is infection with a bacterium called helicobacter pylori. With better sanitation the incidence of infection with this agent has decreased. It can be eradicated by combining antibiotics with medication to decrease gastric acidity.

Melanoma and non-melanoma skin cancers

Melanoma is rare but deserves discussion because the incidence is rising in white-skinned people all over the world. The highest incidence is in Australia where fair-skinned Europeans have migrated to live under a hot sun. In fact, the incidence is higher the closer fair-skinned people live to the equator. Unlike other skin cancers, such as squamous cell cancers, melanoma does not follow a distribution on the body that mirrors sun exposure. In black-skinned people melanomas usually appear on depigmented areas such as the soles of the feet. It has a high incidence in people who work inside, suggesting that intermittent intense exposure is more part of the cause than the continuous exposure that causes other types of skin cancer. The incidence could be expected to increase if phenomena like the enlarged hole in the ozone layer of the atmosphere continue.

Melanoma can be associated with a family history of melanoma and some families have multiple pigmented moles on their skins which could become cancerous. A fair complexion, blue eyes and fair or red hair increase the risk of acquiring the disease.

Lymphomas

There are many distinct types of these cancers but overall they are only the seventh most common type of cancer. Population-based studies have suggested different causative factors from those we have seen for the solid cancers studied so far.

Hodgkin's disease

One member of this family, Hodgkin's disease, named for Thomas Hodgkin who first described it, has two incidence peaks. The first is in young adulthood and the second is an increase in older age in common with many other cancers. This pattern is reminiscent of polio or infections with the virus that causes glandular fever. This led to the theory that early exposure to an infectious agent builds up immunity but, if this does not occur, later exposure could trigger Hodgkin's disease. Support for this comes from the observations that link Hodgkin's disease with a protected childhood environment, higher social class and living in a more affluent country. Childhood infections in people with early onset Hodgkin's disease tended to have been of later onset, and higher concentrations of the antibodies to the Ebstein-Barr virus, the cause of glandular fever, have been found.

Some odd associations with Hodgkin's disease have surfaced from epidemiological studies. A higher incidence in agricultural workers and wood workers has been reported, but not satisfactorily explained.

Non-Hodgkin's lymphomas

Although it has always seemed strange to me that a group of diseases is called by what they are not, non-Hodgkin's lymphomas represent all the lymphomas that don't have the features of Hodgkin's disease under the microscope. These lymphomas are on the increase in most places in the world. One distinct aggressive form, called Burkitt's lymphoma, occurs predominantly in children in Africa and is associated with exposure to the Ebstein-Barr virus.

With the other types of non-Hodgkin's lymphomas, most of the factors that are important in other cancers, such as smoking or diet, do not seem to be related to lymphomas. What does seem to be important is suppression of the immune system. Patients who are taking immunosuppressive drugs after organ transplants have a markedly elevated risk. AIDS patients, whose disease depresses their immune systems, rare genetic diseases where the immune system functions poorly (and children need to be isolated in protected environments) and diseases like rheumatoid arthritis, where the body's immune system acts against itself, are all associated with an increase in the likelihood of developing lymphoma.

Leukaemias

Leukaemias are cancers of white blood cells, produced in the bone marrow and then circulating in high numbers in the blood. Childhood leukaemias are quite different from adult leukaemias and the success in treating them has decreased the death rate from this disease quite significantly. The strongest evidence for a cause of leukaemia—exposure to radiation—has been gathered by monitoring the victims of the atomic bombs dropped on Hiroshima and Nagasaki. The evidence for exposure to lower-dose radiation, such as from x-rays on pregnant mothers or radon gas or exposure to electromagnetic fields from the environment, has been less certain. There has been evidence that some occupational exposures to chemicals such as benzene may constitute a risk factor, and we have already discussed cytotoxic drug exposure being linked with the later development of leukaemias. Links with infectious agents have been strongest in linking a T-cell leukaemia-lymphoma with a retrovirus HTLV 1.

Kaposi's sarcoma

I finish with this disease because it underlines the usefulness of epidemiological observation in disease discovery. Kaposi's sarcoma was originally described in 1872 by Moritz Kaposi as slow-growing purplish nodules classically seen on the legs of elderly eastern European Jews and men from around the Mediterranean Sea. A more aggressive and widespread form of the disease had been recorded in Africa, occurring in younger patients and involving internal organs. Patients who are immunosuppressed after organ transplants could also develop this cancer.

In 1981 a new association was found when young homosexual men in the United States were seen to have an aggressive form of Kaposi's sarcoma together with lymphomas and rare infections, such as pneumocystis pneumonia, that usually occurred only in immunosuppressed patients. This observed grouping led researchers to believe that a new disease causing immunosuppression had begun. The disease became known as the acquired immunodeficiency syndrome or AIDS. Its viral cause was discovered later but doctors were alerted to its presence as a result of the changes observed in the patterns of disease across a population.

SUMMARY

Cancer registries collect details of cancer incidence and mortality and provide us with information about how cancer behaves across whole populations of people. Epidemiological studies can analyse this information and point to the causes of cancer by looking at differences in its behaviour in different populations. We discussed the results of such studies as they applied to the most common types of cancer.

7

Notable cancers

> I've done considerble in the doctoring way in my time.
> Layin' on o' hands is my best holt for cancer, and paraly-
> sis, and sich things; and I k'n tell a fortune pretty good,
> when I've got somebody along to find out the facts for
> me . . .
>
> —*Mark Twain,* The Adventures of Huckleberry Finn, *1884*

Although it takes a large textbook to give details of every cancer, I want to look at specific issues that patients raise about the management of common cancers, and use these to illustrate principles that are common to most cancers. We'll begin with the solid tumours, which are grouped together to distinguish them from the haematological cancers such as lymphomas, myeloma and leukaemia. Why don't we start from the top?

BRAIN TUMOURS

Although cancers arising from the brain are rare in adults they are second to leukaemias in causing cancer deaths in children.

Patients commonly present with headaches which are characteristically worse in the morning and improve as the day goes on. This headache is often due to swelling of the brain, or cerebral oedema, around the tumour. The pressure builds up overnight but the fluid can redistribute on rising.

A small tumour can do a lot of damage in the brain. First, there are a lot of vital nervous system structures close together and, second, the bony skull confines the brain so that any growth increases the pressure on the brain. The symptoms can be general—drowsiness, headache, nausea, seizures, changes in the ability to concentrate. They can also be specific, depending on which part of the brain is affected. Patients may present with weakness, changes in sensation, problems with vision or speech or changes in personality.

The diagnosis is easily made with CT scans or MRI scans which may suggest the need for a biopsy to tell the type of cancer. The definitive treatment is surgery. This will work better in less aggressive cancers where all can be removed without excessive damage to the normal brain. Surgery can be supplemented by radiotherapy which is also used to control aggressive disease that is either inoperable or returns after operation.

Special techniques can be used to implant radioactive sources into a tumour to give high local doses to the tumour while sparing the surrounding brain. Stereotactic radiosurgery, which focuses a radiotherapy beam on a small area, may be used to treat small deep-seated cancers. Chemotherapy is important in childhood brain cancers but has limited use in adults. In aggressive cancers that have been treated with surgery and radiotherapy, further control can be achieved with a combination of drugs (e.g. PCV, procarbazine, lomustine and vincristine) but often only for a few months.

The initial symptoms are often controlled with corticosteroid tablets, particularly dexamethasone, which can reduce the brain swelling around the cancer. Drugs to control seizures and symptom control of pain and nausea may also be required.

155

HEAD AND NECK CANCER

The term 'head and neck cancer' brings together a range of cancers from the mouth to the back of the nose and throat and down to the larynx, or voice box. They are all lined by the same type of cell, the squamous cell, which accounts for most of the cancers in the region. Smoking cigarettes and drinking alcohol is the major risk factor for developing these cancers.

The extent of disease is determined by CT scans and having a look, under anaesthetic, with an endoscope. In general, the mainstay of treatment has been surgery to remove the primary cancer and the draining lymph nodes in the neck. Repairing the defect left by trying to remove all the tumour often requires grafts of flaps of tissue rotated from other areas. Removal of the larynx can mean loss of speech and a tracheostomy or breathing hole in the windpipe. With special techniques or mechanical voice synthesisers, speech can be restored.

Radiation therapy is often used as an adjuvant to surgery to improve local control. For small cancers, radiotherapy can be curative and should be considered as an alternative to surgery that may allow preservation of the larynx and vocal cords, although this may need to be balanced with radiation side effects such as a persistently dry mouth. Chemotherapy with cisplatin and 5 fluorouracil can palliate advanced disease or be used together with the other treatments.

The interesting fact about head and neck cancers is that they tend to remain local and recur locally. Although they can spread to other organs, such as the lungs, most of the problems associated with them occur locally. To improve local control, combinations of all types of treatments have been tried. Currently, there is much interest in the potential for radiotherapy and chemotherapy given together to improve the outcome.

LUNG CANCER

We think of lung cancer in two different categories: small cell lung cancer and non-small cell lung cancer. They behave quite differently. We consider small cell lung cancer a systemic disease. It represents about 25 per cent of lung cancers. It is rarely localised but spreads via the bloodstream early in its natural history. It can present with symptoms common to all lung cancers, such as breathlessness, chest pain or cough, sometimes with blood in the sputum. It may also present with symptoms from sites to where it has spread. Small cell lung cancer can produce hormones that give symptoms remote from the cancer. These can include everything from retaining fluid in the body to weakness and skin rashes.

Small cell lung cancer is very responsive to chemotherapy, such as cisplatin and etoposide, but relapses again. Even with disease that is limited to the chest and responds completely to chemotherapy, the average survival is only 18 months, and only 5–10 per cent of patients survive for five years and are considered cured. Survival may be improved a little by irradiating the main site of disease in the chest. Some relapses occur in the brain even if all the rest of the disease has responded. This suggests that the chemotherapy may not penetrate the brain as effectively as other areas. Irradiating the brain can prevent relapse there but does not improve survival and has side effects of its own.

Non-small cell lung cancers include several different types of cancer which tend to remain localised to the lung for longer in their natural history and are thus potentially curable by surgery. If localised to the lung without spread to the lymph glands in the centre of the chest then aggressive surgery is warranted. This may involve removal of part of a lung or the whole of a lung if the individual is fit enough to survive with one lung.

For very early disease, five-year survival rates of 45 per cent have been reported. For more extensive disease that can be encompassed in a radiation field without excessive damage to surrounding normal tissue full-dose radiotherapy alone will cure 5–10 per cent.

Recent research into the treatment of disease that involves some nodes in the centre of the chest on the same side as the cancer suggests that combining the treatment modalities of surgery, radiotherapy and even chemotherapy can improve survival. Radiotherapy in shorter courses can be very effective in controlling the symptoms of pain or cough if a cancer is blocking a bronchus. Local techniques where radiation sources can be placed inside an airway have been useful for local control of the cancer.

Blocked airways can also be relieved by use of a laser during bronchoscopy or the insertion of expanding sleeves into a narrow area which spring open and stent the airway open to counter the compression from a cancer.

In widespread disease chemotherapy has been disappointing. In the last few years, however, more drugs with activity against non-small cell lung cancers have been identified. The taxanes, gemcitabine and navelbine are being combined with platinums to give response rates of more than 50 per cent. Unfortunately, however, although there have been some gains, the improvement in survival in most trials is only weeks to months. Quality of life questions, particularly while on chemotherapy, become important here.

Like small cell lung cancers, non-small cell lung cancers can have remote effects that are not due to metastases. Squamous cell lung cancers can produce a hormone which elevates the blood calcium and causes dryness, drowsiness and constipation— these can be difficult to distinguish from symptoms that are directly due to the tumour. This situation can easily be reversed with simple treatments and so should be investigated. Another remote effect which seems odd is the so-called clubbing or enlarging of the fingernails or toenails, often associated with painful forearms or legs.

A feature of lung cancer which it shares with many cancers is that outcome and survival depend very much on how well a patient is at the time of diagnosis. This is independent of the treatment used and can guide the decision about whether treatment will be worthwhile. Patients who have lost more than 10 per cent of their body weight in the months before presentation would be expected to survive only half the length of time of those who have maintained their weight. Those who are bedridden will do badly and aggressive treatment will not be helpful.

CANCERS OF THE DIGESTIVE SYSTEM

The digestive tract consists of the oesophagus, or gullet, the stomach, the small bowel, and the large bowel which ends at the anus. The liver and the pancreas secrete digestive juices into the small bowel.

Oesophageal cancer

This disease is five times as common in males and is associated with smoking in the West and nitrosamines in the food in the East. The patient usually presents with difficulty in swallowing and weight loss. The disease can easily be demonstrated by swallowing barium and taking x-ray pictures, or by a direct look with an endoscope.

Once surgery was the only approach but the expected five-year survival, even if it looked as if all had been cleared, was only one in five. Now, combining treatments has improved the outcome. There is increasing evidence from clinical trials that giving radiotherapy and chemotherapy together prior to surgery improves the outcome.

For patients who are too sick for aggressive treatment, relief may be obtained by lasering the obstructing tumour through an endoscope. Failing that, patients can be fed by using an endoscope to position a feeding tube that will go through the abdominal wall into the stomach (often called a PEG for percutaneous endoscopic gastrostomy).

Stomach

Cancers of the body of the stomach are becoming less common but those near the junction with the oesophagus are increasing, for reasons that are not clear. Most patients present complaining of indigestion and weight loss, although symptoms may be more like those of an ulcer with pain and bleeding.

Primarily, the treatment is surgical. In this cancer, however, there is no evidence that additional or adjuvant chemotherapy alters survival. More advanced local disease can be palliated with radiotherapy. Chemotherapy is used for locally advanced or widespread cancers. Here the news is becoming more encouraging. Newer multi-agent chemotherapy regimens such as ECF (epirubicin, cisplatin, 5 fluorouracil) are beginning to show higher rates of complete remission, which then gives a chance that the disease will not return.

Large bowel cancer

Cancers of the small bowel are rare but, as discussed earlier, there is a high incidence of large bowel cancers. Although often regarded together as colorectal cancer, the rectum at the end of the large bowel is treated differently from the rest of the large bowel or colon. The bowel is lined with gland-forming cells and the cancers of these cells are called adenocarcinomas. At the outer end of the large bowel is the anus, which is different again because it is lined with squamous cells, like those that make up the covering of the skin outside.

Unless detected by screening, colon cancers present differently depending on which end of the bowel is affected. Cancers of the right side of the colon tend to grow for longer without symptoms and present with a slow blood loss which causes the patient to be pale with anaemia. They can also cause abdominal pain or bloating. On the left side, cancers nearer to the end of the bowel are most likely to cause bright red blood loss with bowel motions, or bowel obstruction with cramping pains. Both may be suspected simply by a change in bowel habits—constipation, diarrhoea or alternation between the two. With very advanced disease, patients may present with symptoms of the metastases which are usually in the liver.

Colon cancer is curable by surgery if diagnosed early. The best guide to the likelihood of cure is gained after the removal of the cancer when the pathologist can tell us how far the cancer has penetrated through the bowel wall. For patients whose cancer is confined to the inner lining of the bowel, 95 per cent could expect to be alive at five years. If it has penetrated through the wall, the figure drops to below 25 per cent and, if widespread, the figure is 5 per cent.

Over the last few years, large clinical trials have found there is a survival benefit to offering chemotherapy in addition to the surgery for those patients with tumours that have penetrated the bowel wall. Essentially, the same drugs are used as for advanced disease. The survival benefit of giving six months of chemotherapy with a regimen such as 5 fluorouracil and leucovorin continues to be apparent over many years follow-up.

Follow-up after the operation will involve periodic checks by looking with a colonoscope and removing any suspicious polyps. Blood tests include CEA (carcinoembryonic antigen) which can be a marker of relapse in those cancers that produce it.

Surgery is the mainstay of treatment for rectal cancer. In low cancers there may not be enough bowel to join together and a colostomy is created, where the bowel empties into a bag worn on the abdominal wall. In this setting it is permanent but, sometimes, particularly in treating a colon cancer that has caused obstruction and the bowel has swollen, such an opening may have to be created temporarily and later reversed.

Radiotherapy plays a role in the adjuvant therapy of rectal cancer. The rectum is fixed and localised whereas the colon hangs in the abdomen on a membrane and can move freely, making it difficult to irradiate. The advantage in local control of irradiation after surgery for rectal cancer must be balanced by possible damage to the bowel and bladder, causing long-term symptoms. With newer techniques there are fewer side effects. Recently, it has been suggested that the best use of radiotherapy in this setting is to give it before the operation. More clinical trials are being performed to investigate this approach. Additional chemotherapy can be useful, as with colon cancer, but the best combination of treatments is still the subject of ongoing research.

For widespread colorectal cancer, chemotherapy is an option for control of symptoms. Until recently there was only one drug, 5 fluorouracil, on which all treatments were based. The absence of new drugs led to some innovative attempts to improve the response to 5 fluorouracil, which usually achieves meaningful shrinkage of the cancer in less than one in five patients. One of the actions of 5 fluorouracil is to block an enzyme necessary for making RNA. Of many agents tried to improve the ability of 5 fluorouracil to do this, leucovorin has stood the test of time and is now given in combination with 5 fluorouracil.

Another approach was based on the fact that 5 fluorouracil only stays in the blood for a short time. With the development of small portable pumps that patients can easily carry with them clipped to the belt like a portable radio, and implanted devices that can provide access to a vein in the chest so that the arms can be kept free, 5 fluorouracil can be given as a prolonged infusion, over many months if well tolerated. If patients have disease confined to the liver, similar technology allows drugs to be given directly into the liver at high concentrations without damaging the normal liver cells because there are two sources of blood supply to the liver.

With all this, less than one-third of patients respond and there is little or no impact on survival. Some responders may have their disease well controlled but chemotherapy is not curative and so some patients choose to have the symptoms of their bowel cancer treated without chemotherapy. New drugs such as the camptothecan analogues and others that specifically inhibit the same enzyme as 5 fluorouracil seek to improve the outcome with chemotherapy for metastatic disease.

Although rare, carcinoma of the anus deserves a mention because it is a good example of research providing more options for treatment. Surgery had been the main treatment but this often removed the lower part of the bowel and left patients with a colostomy. A combination of chemotherapy (mitomycin C and 5 fluorouracil) and radiotherapy has had such promising results that many patients can avoid major surgery.

Liver cancer

Liver cancer is rare, but most patients who are diagnosed with the disease survive for less than a year. Surgery is the treatment required. The liver has such amazing reserve that up to 80 per cent of it can be removed and the remaining liver will sustain the function as long as it is healthy. The problem is that primary liver cancer occurs after hepatitis B infection, iron overload in the liver or alcoholic liver disease so the often aggressive treatment is not an option. Because of the dual blood supply to the liver, attempts to block the main liver artery that feeds the tumour can achieve some control. Drugs can be given into the liver or systemically but they have little success. Liver transplant has been tried for very localised cancers, but applies only to a highly selected and fit group of patients and must still be regarded as experimental.

Cancer of the pancreas

Most patients present with this cancer when it is beyond surgical treatment. Of the one in five who may be suitable for surgery, only one in five will be cured by the large operation. Radiotherapy and chemotherapy may add to the local control but, for more widespread disease, no chemotherapy has been curative and shrinkage of the cancer is achieved only rarely. This is just the type of cancer where innovative approaches and new drugs with different targets within the cell are required. This is the thrust of clinical research programs with this cancer.

163

FEMALE CANCERS

Many cancers of the female reproductive organs will be responsive to the female hormones because the organ from which they are derived is under the control of these chemical messengers produced from glands at other sites in the body. This provides a further avenue for attacking these cancers.

Breast cancer

Although breast cancer can occur in males it is rare, but breast cancer is very common in women. Earlier chapters discussed screening, diagnosis and epidemiology and I now want to explain what choices are available for the management of breast cancer.

Surgery is the first treatment considered when a breast lump is found. There are essentially two treatment choices. Either a mastectomy is performed where all the breast tissue is removed, or only the lump is removed and the rest of the breast is irradiated. The second procedure preserves the breast and large clinical trials have confirmed that the survival outcomes are equivalent. Not every patient is suitable for breast conservation. A large cancer in a small breast would mean a poor cosmetic result. Reconstruction of the breast then becomes an option. In patients with locally advanced disease with a big primary or fixed lymph glands beneath the arm, chemotherapy and radiotherapy may precede surgery to shrink the disease first.

The other surgical procedure considered is to remove the lymph glands from beneath the arm (axilla). The two reasons for doing this are that it removes any breast cancer that has reached the nodes and it also has significance for deciding how the disease is going to behave and whether additional treatment will be necessary. This latter reason for surgery to the axilla is becoming less important. Not so long ago, patients with cancerous glands under the arm were offered additional systemic therapy, those without were not. This was based on the fact that the survival of women with positive nodes was shorter than

164

if glands were not involved, and additional treatment had been shown in clinical trials to improve that survival. However, some node-negative women will benefit from additional therapy. It has been difficult to judge who they are. Some doctors treat all women with adjuvant therapy, others try to pick the node-negative group with the more aggressive disease as evidenced by the size of the primary and various markers on the cell which are demonstrated by the pathologist and correlate with aggressiveness.

There are two types of additional therapy after surgery. Local radiotherapy is given to improve local control and prevent the breast cancer returning locally. Whether it is necessary depends on factors such as the extent of the surgery, the size of the primary, the closeness of the cancer to the surgical margins and the spread to the axillary nodes, which may suggest that other surrounding nodes are involved.

It is more important, however, to prevent distant relapse. We need systemic therapy for that and there are two main choices—hormone treatment and chemotherapy. We want to be aggressive upfront because the disease at this stage can still be cured. We can measure the likelihood of a breast cancer responding to hormone treatment by measuring whether it has receptors for hormones on its surface. Those tumours which are positive for oestrogen and progesterone receptors are more likely to respond to hormone manipulation and have a better outlook. Again, a few years ago, the story was simple. Women who had gone through the menopause were treated with hormones, while those still menstruating were treated with chemotherapy. There followed a series of clinical trials and an analysis, called a meta-analysis, of all the data collected from multiple trials of adjuvant therapy. Adding chemotherapy to hormone therapy in the postmenopausal group appears to add survival benefit. The same may be seen in the premenopausal group but chemotherapy there also interferes with menstrual cycles, which may explain part of its success.

The options for hormone therapy in the premenopausal group include removing the ovaries or using hormone injections or tablets. Tamoxifen, an anti-oestrogen, is the most common tablet given to postmenopausal women.

There are several choices possible for chemotherapy when used in addition to surgery. Overall, the greatest benefit is in the premenopausal group, where there has been a reduction in deaths by up to 25 per cent by ten years. Conventional-dose chemotherapy regimens, which are the same as those used to treat metastatic disease, fall into those containing an anthracycline drug such as doxorubicin and those based on the common regimen CMF (cyclophosphamide, methotrexate and 5 fluorouracil). Current chemotherapy regimens still do poorly with women who have a large number of lymph glands involved under the arm. This is the group, in particular, where high-dose regimens requiring bone marrow or peripheral blood stem cell transplants have been investigated. Early results have been promising, but only in highly selected groups of patients. There are currently several large randomised trials of high-dose against standard-dose therapy that will tell us the place of this treatment.

For widespread disease, either chemotherapy or hormone therapy is used. Widespread breast cancer is incurable, with an average survival of two years. This is a reason for wanting to put so much effort into initial therapy when the disease is still curable. Controlling metastatic disease, however, is important for quality of life. Hormone therapy, which is simple and has few side effects, is preferred but is only useful if the cancer is hormone receptor positive. Many new hormones are becoming available and several different hormones can be tried against responsive cancers. Hormones take some weeks before their effect is seen. Rapidly progressive disease or cancer in vital organs such as the liver or lungs should therefore be treated with chemotherapy, and hormone therapy should be left for disease in structural tissues such as the skin, lymph glands or bones. There are several different well defined drug combinations that are very effective in shrinking breast cancer. The good news is that there is also a number of new agents, particularly the taxanes, that are proving very effective against metastatic disease and are being incorporated into standard treatments. High-dose chemotherapy is also being explored in this setting.

Symptom control can also be aided by radiotherapy, which in short courses is very effective in controlling bone pain. A new class of drugs called the bisphosphonates, some of which are now available in tablet form, can also prevent some of the problems associated with having breast cancer in the bones.

Cancer of the ovary

An interesting characteristic of ovarian cancer is that in most cases it remains confined to the abdomen. Unless it is already known to have spread to distant sites, the initial procedure is an operation by an experienced gynaecological oncologist which serves to make the diagnosis, assess the extent of the disease and cut out as much as possible. With limited disease, this operation may be curative. If the disease has been extensive in the abdomen or if it presents with widespread disease, chemotherapy is used. This therapy is based on the drug cisplatin, traditionally combined with cyclophosphamide but more recently with paclitaxel, as paclitaxel had initially proved useful after cisplatin failures. In advanced disease, complete responses can be achieved in one-third of patients but, although control can be achieved for a couple of years, the disease usually returns and the average survival is around three years.

CA 125 is a marker that can be used to follow the progress of those ovarian cancers which produce it. This technique can be used to monitor the response to chemotherapy as a supplement to scans and may signal relapse before visible disease is apparent.

Cancer of the uterus

Screening for cancer of the cervix allows changes prior to cancer—or at least very early cancers—to be detected. These can be cured surgically, often by hysterectomy. When the disease is more advanced in the pelvis, local radiotherapy, often combined with chemotherapy, becomes part of the available treatments. For widespread disease, regimens containing cisplatin are often used.

Cancer of the lining of the uterus, endometrial cancer, is seen in patients at or past the menopause. It is often diagnosed because of abnormal bleeding. Early disease can be cured by surgery alone, which usually means removing the uterus, tubes and ovaries as well as sampling the surrounding tissue to determine the risk of recurrence. High-risk patients may receive a combination of surgery and radiotherapy. For widespread disease, hormone therapy with MPA (medroxyprogesterone acetate) or tamoxifen, much as used in breast cancer, can control the disease for several months. Chemotherapy can achieve similar results using drugs such as doxorubicin. I will return to endometrial cancer when discussing prevention since there is a concern that long-term use of tamoxifen may increase the incidence of this cancer.

MALE CANCERS

Cancers of the male organs associated with reproduction have an important place in discussions about cancer. Prostate cancer is important because it is so common and testicular cancer is important because it is so curable.

Prostate cancer

The dilemma of screening for prostate cancer is discussed in Chapter 4. Does very early low-grade disease need treatment? There are more dilemmas. If we have localised disease in the prostate that should be treated, what is the best treatment? The options lie between surgery to remove the prostate and radiotherapy. Surgery requires that the patient be fit enough for an operation, but can be associated with incontinence and impotence. Radiotherapy avoids the immediate problems of an operation but can also result in loss of continence and gradual impotence, as well as irritation of the bladder or large bowel. One practice has been to operate on patients under 70 years and irradiate older or less fit patients. Surgery has been improved by the use of nerve-sparing operations which can reduce the rate of sexual problems and incontinence. Radiotherapy has improved in its ability to irradiate the prostate more precisely and spare the surrounding tissues. Newer techniques involve implanting the prostate with radioactive seeds or implanting wires for local therapy. These will need further testing against external radiotherapy. The survival rates for early-stage disease have been quoted at 90 per cent and 85 per cent for surgery and radiotherapy respectively, and both treatment modalities are reasonable options. While there may be a benefit in local control for adding radiotherapy to surgery if there is still at least microscopic disease left, it is doubtful whether this impacts on survival. Adding hormone treatment immediately to surgery in locally more aggressive cancers may also not significantly alter survival, but more information from clinical trials would be useful here.

For advanced disease, hormone therapy is the therapy of choice. There are several different ways of switching off the stimulus that male hormones have on the prostate. The gold standard treatment was to remove the testicles. Of equal efficacy is to give hormones called LHRH (luteinising hormone releasing hormone) analogues. Initially, these mimic the actions of the hormones released from the brain that eventually lead to stimulation of the production of the male hormone, testosterone, from the testicles, but quickly exhaust the ability to cause that stimulation and turn off the testosterone. These hormones need to be given by monthly injection although longer-acting forms are now available. Other hormones block the male hormone production directly. They can be given with LHRH analogues to block the initial release of testosterone. Randomised trials, however, have shown no survival benefit in giving them after removal of the testicles and thus make patients uncomfortable by causing diarrhoea.

Once a cancer progresses after the first hormone treatment the response to a further hormone treatment is limited. Unfortunately, unlike breast cancer, there are no good chemotherapy options for prostate cancer, despite ongoing clinical trials. Since bone is often the site of spread it is difficult to assess response since bones take a long time to heal. If chemotherapy is to be tried it should be added to the hormone treatment that the patient was taking when progression occurred, since hormones may still control some hormone-sensitive parts of the cancer. This is unlike failures on chemotherapy where the new drug replaces the old because the progressive disease is resistant.

Since a large proportion of patients who develop widespread disease have bone metastases and bone pain, radiotherapy is a very good option for relief. There are several ways this can be achieved. Small areas of severe pain can be irradiated. Often it only takes a few doses to relieve the pain. For more widespread pain, single half-body doses can be given with relief often following within a day. Another alternative is to inject isotopes such as strontium which is taken up by the bone and gives widespread local irradiation. Pain relief should be given and often steroids will assist in the control of symptoms.

PSA tests are used to follow the progress of the disease and may detect breakthrough of hormone treatment long before clinical symptoms are manifest. Patients who are being followed up post surgery, or while on steroids, are very interested in their PSA levels to see if their disease is being kept under control. They need to understand, however, that once they have widespread disease the PSA becomes less relevant than the symptoms, which become the arbiter of whether to treat.

Testicular cancer

Testicular cancer is the shining example of the ability of chemotherapy to cure a widespread solid cancer. It also has very sensitive markers of its presence, which can be measured in the bloodstream and used to follow the progress of the disease and guide treatment. At least one of the markers, either αFP (alpha fetoprotein) or βHCG (beta human chorionic gonadotrophin) will be elevated in 80 per cent of testicular cancers.

Testicular cancers are divided into seminomas, which represent about 40 per cent of the total number and have no elevated markers (occasionally βHCG may be raised), and the others which are called non-seminomas (just like non-small cell lung cancers and non-Hodgkin's lymphomas where all the other types are grouped together because they behave similarly). Non-seminomas can have a mixture of cells, evident because often both markers, each of which comes from a different cell type, are raised.

The treatment of cancer confined to the testicle is surgical removal. The testicle is removed through a small cut in the groin, not through the scrotal sac. With seminomas, postoperative radiotherapy is used to treat the lymph nodes in the abdomen where any cells escaping from the testicle would travel. The disease is very sensitive to radiotherapy and the cure rate is high. (It would probably be just as high with additional chemotherapy but radiotherapy is the historical treatment and who can argue with success?) Chemotherapy is used if the disease has spread to the lymph nodes and is too bulky for radiotherapy.

For non-seminomas there are several choices. In some centres, patients have removal of the testicle and the draining lymph nodes, just to be certain of cure. Other centres remove the testicle and watch patients closely with regular blood tests for markers and chest x-rays for two years. Yet again, some doctors try to pick the worst cancers—those that have invaded blood vessels or the wall of the testicle—and treat with chemotherapy after surgery. The reason for such a diversity of early treatment is that if the disease does return after the initial surgery there is a 90 per cent chance of it responding to chemotherapy. It is also possible for relapse to be diagnosed very early because markers may rise before any cancer becomes visible.

For disease that has spread, the treatment is chemotherapy. The drug that has made all the difference to cure of testicular cancer is cisplatin. The PEB (cisplatin, etoposide and bleomycin) regimen achieves complete disappearance of the cancer in more than 90 per cent of cases. If the cancer does not return within two years of treatment it is likely the patient has been cured.

The likelihood of disease responding depends on how much cancer there is. At the best end of the scale, the markers are elevated but there is no visible cancer. It should be noted that if markers are elevated prior to operating on the testicle the operation will not cause an instant fall to normal—it can take several days to weeks for the markers to be cleared from the blood. If there is cancer left after three or four courses of PEB it can be removed or second-line chemotherapy given. High-dose chemotherapy with bone marrow rescue has been used successfully for some patients who had relapsed after initially responding to chemotherapy.

Occasionally, a testicular cancer can appear outside the testicle in the chest or abdomen, without a lump in the testicle. These are treated with the same chemotherapy, but tend not to respond as well as their testicular counterparts.

Most of the research in testicular cancer has been to make the highly successful chemotherapy more tolerable. There is also scope for improving the outcome of the worst cancers.

CANCERS OF THE URINARY TRACT

To complete the urinary tract, we need to consider cancers of the kidney and bladder.

Kidney cancer

Kidney cancer can present quite late with symptoms of pain, blood in the urine and a lump in the abdomen, or generalised symptoms such as weight loss. The main treatment is surgical removal since we can function quite well with only one kidney. Once the disease has spread, however, there is no chemotherapy which is effective and so participation in trials of new drugs is offered.

Four in ten patients will have disease that has spread. In that case there is no benefit for survival in removing the kidney. If the cancer is causing symptoms it can either be removed or

172

its blood supply can be blocked. Even with metastatic disease, there is an enormous variation in the pace of progression, ranging from death within months to patients surviving more than a decade. Kidney cancer is one of those cancers where spontaneous disappearance of metastases without treatment has been observed.

Cancer of the bladder

The lining of the urinary tract from the outlet of the kidney to the bladder is the same type of cell, called a transitional cell, and this is where the commonest cancer arises. The presenting symptom is often blood in the urine which is investigated by looking into the bladder with a cystoscope. If the cancer remains confined to this lining, the small growths can be killed by burning them off through a cystoscope. Regular checks are needed since it must be assumed that the whole lining of the bladder is affected by the changes that caused the cancer. For multiple cancers, in addition to removing them, chemotherapy or BCG can be instilled into the bladder to help control the disease.

For cancers that penetrate deeper into the wall of the bladder, removal of the bladder is required. The urine then has to be diverted and collected in a bag worn on the abdomen, or an artificial 'bladder' created using a loop of bowel. Radiotherapy can be used as a local treatment to the bladder and surrounding lymph glands, and results can be improved by giving it with cisplatin. The role of chemotherapy as an adjuvant after surgery is still being defined but with better chemotherapy for advanced disease this approach holds promise. The introduction of multi-agent chemotherapy like the MVAC (methotrexate, vinblastine, doxorubicin, cisplatin) regimen has made some cures of widespread disease possible with approximately one in six patients surviving five years.

SKIN CANCER AND MELANOMA

Melanoma is the most aggressive of the skin cancers because of its propensity to spread throughout the body. Melanomas tend to grow across the surface of the skin before they grow downwards. The likelihood of widespread disease increases with the depth of the melanoma when it is removed. It is essential, therefore, to remove a melanoma as early in its development as possible. Studies are being done to determine whether the draining lymph glands should be removed as well but it is not routinely recommended.

The main treatment for melanoma is surgical, whether it be of the primary or of a secondary deposit in lymph nodes or elsewhere. An attempt should be made to leave the patient with no evidence of disease. Adding chemotherapy to surgery has been of no benefit but there are promising early results of using adjuvant immunotherapy with tumour vaccines or interferon. In widespread disease, chemotherapy with dacarbazine has a limited role, shrinking only 20 per cent of tumours, and usually only for a short time. One novel approach has been used for those patients where multiple deposits of melanoma are confined to a limb. The blood supply to the limb can be isolated and high-dose chemotherapy given into the artery and drained from the vein, so that it can't affect the rest of the body. Investigational approaches in widespread melanoma using immunotherapy alone or with chemotherapy are the focus for current researchers.

Non-melanoma skin cancers are the most common cancers of humans. They are also the most curable because they tend to remain localised for their lifespan. This means that the treatment is to remove them. The old adage 'if in doubt chop it out' is probably a reasonable approach to avoid the risk of a large local area of destruction or the occasional skin cancer that will metastasise. In most cases, though, it is easy to distinguish cancers from benign spots. For cosmetically sensitive areas, it is worth knowing that many skin cancers can also be cured by radiotherapy.

LYMPHOMAS AND LEUKAEMIAS

The haematological cancers arising from cells in the bone marrow or lymphoid system usually require systemic treatment and are the most sensitive of malignancies to chemotherapy.

Hodgkin's and non-Hodgkin's lymphomas

We have discussed these cancers in earlier chapters. Both are malignancies of the lymph nodes with several types distinguished from each other by their appearance under the microscope. They tend to spread along the chains of lymph glands, Hodgkin's disease staying more in the midline, non-Hodgkin's disease involving more peripheral glands. The extent of disease is expressed in terms of whether it is confined to a local group or groups of glands on one or both sides of the diaphragm (which separates the chest from the abdomen) or whether it has spread to other organs. The specific generalised symptoms, called B symptoms, of weight loss of greater than 10 per cent, fever, and drenching night sweats are also taken into consideration because they worsen the outlook. Some novel symptoms such as itch and pain after drinking alcohol have also been associated with lymphomas.

Hodgkin's disease localised to one side of the diaphragm and without general symptoms can be cured in most patients with radiotherapy. All the nodes can be covered in radiotherapy fields. A mantle field, likened to a cloak, covers the nodes of the neck, under the arms and central chest above the diaphragm. An inverted Y, covering the chain of nodes in the centre of the abdomen and then down into each groin, covers those below the diaphragm.

More widespread disease requires chemotherapy. The original regimen for Hodgkin's disease, MOPP (nitrogen mustard, vincristine, procarbazine and prednisolone), was one of the initial multi-agent chemotherapy regimens designed so that the drugs did not have overlapping side effects. It is highly effective, with 84 per cent of patients achieving complete disappearance of disease and over half being disease-free more than twenty years later. MOPP is still used but other regimens such as ABVD (doxorubicin, bleomycin, vinblastine, dacarbazine) provide alternative treatment with different side effects.

Non-Hodgkin's lymphomas are graded by the pattern of the disease under the microscope and the use of special stains into low, intermediate and high grades, which should correlate with their clinical behaviour. Low-grade disease is not regarded as curable and grumbles along for many years. We often see lymph glands swell and shrink without any treatment at all. We only treat if the swollen glands are causing a problem. If it is a local problem, radiotherapy can be used. If the lymphoma is wide-spread we use chemotherapy, often starting with tablets of chlorambucil with prednisolone. Sometimes, low-grade disease can change during the course of its history into higher grades and has to be treated accordingly. Research is directed towards finding whether very aggressive approaches such as high-dose therapy and stem cell transplant could cure this disease.

The higher grades of lymphoma are treated like widespread disease even if they appear localised. They can, for example, involve the bone marrow as well as the lymph glands and other organs. Designing a new chemotherapy combination also appears to involve thinking up a clever acronym and the tried and true chemotherapy for intermediate-grade lymphoma is known as CHOP (cyclophosphamide, doxorubicin, vincristine and predni-solone—the H and O refer to alternative names for the drugs). Complete responses are seen in up to 60 per cent of patients and at least half will remain disease-free, most relapses occurring in the first two years.

High-grade lymphomas are treated more intensively with chemotherapy regimens approximating those used for leukae-mias. Because high-grade lymphomas tend to involve the lining of the brain and spinal cord, drugs are injected into the spinal fluid as well as into the veins as part of the treatment.

Lymphomas are increased in AIDS patients. The lymphomas in this group tend to be more aggressive and present more often with organ involvement, particularly the brain.

Given that such a high percentage of patients with lympho-mas are cured, most of the research involving lymphomas involves trying to give more intense therapy using high-dose chemotherapy and bone marrow or peripheral blood stem cell transplants. Often the bone marrow or stem cells can be har-vested from a patient before high-dose therapy. Other possible sources of bone marrow are matched donors who have had their bone marrow cells typed, much like cross-matching blood. Suitable matches can be hard to find outside patients' relatives. High-dose therapy has been shown to be more successful than conventional-dose chemotherapy in salvaging patients who have relapsed after successful treatment initially.

Leukaemias

Leukaemias are malignancies of the white blood cells produced in the bone marrow. They are divided into acute or chronic according to the time course of the disease and are classified by the cell type that has become malignant. Acute myeloid leukaemia is the most common in adults. It requires intensive chemotherapy—called induction chemotherapy—to try to eradicate the malignant cells in the bone marrow. The chemotherapy is based on cytosine arabinoside and anthracyclines. The biggest problem in treating leukaemia is the length of time that the blood counts are down after intense therapy. The two main complications are severe infections, often with nasty organisms, and bleeding. White cell growth factors such as G-CSF may be helpful here. Current treatments can achieve complete responses 65–85 per cent of the time and the good news is that 15–30 per cent of patients can be cured. Unfortunately, the induction chemotherapy is usually not enough to achieve prolonged control and further courses of similar chemotherapy are given to consolidate the response. Following that, outpatient maintenance chemotherapy can be used. The spinal fluid can be involved in leukaemia and may require chemotherapy to be injected into it.

It is not surprising that high-dose therapy with bone marrow transplants from normal donors has been tried in acute leukaemia. It is used particularly if relapse occurs after initial treatment.

Acute lymphatic leukaemia is treated with different regimens but similar principles in terms of aggressive induction treatment and then maintenance chemotherapy. There is a need for prevention of relapse in and around the brain by treatment with chemotherapy into the spinal fluid and irradiation of the brain. Three of every four patients will achieve a complete response and about half of all patients will still be alive at five years.

Chronic myeloid leukaemia has a well defined chromosome abnormality, called the Philadelphia chromosome, by which the malignant cells are identified. It has three phases. There is a chronic phase which lasts for four to five years where most of the symptoms are general, like weight loss and fever. There follows an accelerated phase over six months when the white cell counts increase rapidly, then a so-called blast crisis, when chronic leukaemia transforms into an acute leukaemia. The chronic phase can be controlled by chemotherapy tablets like hydroxyurea or busulphan, but little is successful in the acute phases. Interferon may achieve durable complete remissions in the chronic phase. High-dose chemotherapy with bone marrow transplantation has been suggested to attempt to cure patients with chronic myeloid leukaemia in the chronic phase. To have the best chance of success, chemotherapy would need to be used early in the disease. The side effects of high-dose therapy, including the chance of death, need to be balanced against the likelihood of long-term survival given that current treatment has patients living for several years.

Chronic lymphocytic leukaemia is often picked up incidentally on blood tests. It does not require immediate treatment. It may cause general symptoms such as fever or fatigue, or the patient may experience an increasing number of infections. When it is associated with lymph node enlargement it behaves very much like low-grade lymphoma and can be treated with similar drugs, such as chlorambucil and prednisolone, or newer agents such as fludarabine. Rarely, transformation to an acute leukaemia can occur. Much of the treatment is directed at preventing infections, using immunoglobulins and pneumococcal vaccines, and giving blood products as needed to relieve symptoms.

Myeloma

Myeloma is a malignancy of the plasma cells of the bone marrow. These are responsible for making the proteins called gamma globulins which help fight infection. In myeloma, high levels of an abnormal protein are produced, part of which is excreted with the urine as Bence Jones proteins. Myeloma is often seen to produce multiple holes in bones. It can present with symptoms from any of these—specifically anaemias, infections or bone pain and high blood calciums. Kidney failure can also occur. The long-used treatment is melphalan and prednisolone tablets which gain control of the symptoms and decrease the level of the abnormal protein produced. There are very few complete responses and life expectancy is two to three years. More intensive intravenous chemotherapy is being tried and it is hoped that high-dose therapy with donor bone marrow transplants will improve the outcome. Symptoms are treated as required. Bone pain responds to anti-inflammatory drugs, radiotherapy and a new class of drugs called bisphosphonates, which have been shown to reduce bone complications in this disease as well as breast cancer.

SARCOMAS

Tumours of the supportive tissues—bone, muscle, fibrous tissues and fat—are called sarcomas. The same treatment principles apply to sarcomas as to carcinomas. Surgery is the main treatment. With osteosarcomas (i.e. sarcomas of bone), amputation is being replaced, where feasible, with surgery that spares the limbs. Radiotherapy may add to local control. Randomised trials have shown that additional chemotherapy adds to survival.

With soft tissue sarcomas, similar extensive surgery should be attempted to remove all the disease if possible. Radiotherapy can improve local control but adjuvant chemotherapy is not routinely used. For metastatic disease, regimens based on doxorubicin and ifosfamide are common. Sarcomas often spread

179

to the lungs. If there are isolated lung lesions, surgical resection can still achieve cure.

Mesothelioma is a specific type of sarcoma appearing on the lining of the lungs or abdomen. It is associated with prior asbestos exposure. It can be difficult to remove entirely by surgery because it is often a sheet of cancer rather than a lump, but reducing the bulk of the disease may improve the control of symptoms. Standard systemic treatments have proved disappointing and so experimental treatments are warranted.

Kaposi's sarcoma in its most aggressive form occurs with AIDS. It is not usually cured but can be controlled with chemotherapy containing doxorubicin. Newer ways of giving doxorubicin include a preparation where it is encapsulated in liposomes—these are fat balls which help to reduce its side effects. Local lesions are also very sensitive to radiotherapy, but treatment must always be placed in the context of what other problems the immunosuppression is causing.

RARE CANCERS

It is beyond the scope of this book to mention all the possible sites of cancers, but similar treatment principles apply to treating local and widespread disease. There are cancers that will have special manifestations such as those of endocrine glands which usually secrete hormones into the body. A cancer of the adrenal gland, for example, may present because of overproduction of adrenal hormones.

Thyroid cancer concentrates iodine and this fact can be used to treat the disease by injecting radioactive iodine which can be taken up by any residual disease after surgery. Many of the rarer cancers may respond poorly to chemotherapy, but decisions can only be made from case reports because there are not enough cases to compare treatments by performing large randomised trials.

CHILDHOOD CANCERS

It is important to realise that, in cancer terms, children are not just small adults. Many of the principles of treatment are similar but there are modifications. For example, radiation to growing bones will stop their development, causing later deformity, and is avoided if possible. In general, the cure rate in childhood cancers is very encouraging.

The most common childhood leukaemia is acute lymphoblastic leukaemia, whereas in adults it is acute myeloid leukaemia. Intensive chemotherapy induction regimens have a remission rate of 90 per cent and include prophylactic treatment to the brain. To maintain the remission maintenance, chemotherapy is given for three years, but 80 per cent of those who successfully complete them will remain disease-free.

The solid tumours are also quite different. Brain tumours are common and can be treated with surgery and radiotherapy as in adults, but multi-agent chemotherapy is more useful than in adults. Kidney cancers are not the same as in adults but present as nephroblastomas or Wilm's tumours and appear at an average age of three and a half years. With aggressive multi-modality treatment using surgery, chemotherapy and radiotherapy as required, these do best of all childhood cancers. Neuroblastomas require a treatment approach that combines chemotherapy and surgery, but has a high cure rate in children under twelve months. Primitive sarcomas are also successfully treated with aggressive combined modality treatment.

CANCER OF UNKNOWN PRIMARY SITE

I conclude with cancers of unknown primary site, to make the point that these are real entities—it's not that we can't be bothered looking or haven't looked hard enough for the primary. They are said to represent 2–10 per cent of all patients presenting with cancer. Even at autopsy, 20–30 per cent of primary sites won't be found. Presumably, the primary is a tiny nest of cells somewhere, causing no symptoms. The primary is unknown if the pathologist cannot identify the organ of origin from a biopsy of one of the metastases, despite the use of special stains and electron micrographs.

The investigation of an unknown primary should not include every possible test. What is important is that we don't miss widespread cancers that are curable such as testicular cancers, easily treatable cancers such as ovarian cancers, breast or prostate cancers and easily diagnosed cancers such as lung cancer when it is clearly visible on a chest x-ray. If there are no symptoms suggesting a primary site and nothing is found on clinical examination, we would perform a chest x-ray and possibly these days a CT of the abdomen and pelvis. Marker studies would be done to look for testicular, prostate, breast and ovarian cancers. Bowel motions and urine are tested for blood. In women, a mammogram and a gynaecological examination are performed. If a head and neck primary is possible because the presenting disease is a lymph node in the neck, then a good ear, nose and throat examination is prudent.

If all this is negative, localised disease is removed or irradiated. Widespread disease can be treated with a broad spectrum chemotherapy regimen which contains drugs appropriate for all the treatable cancers. If the primary site subsequently manifests itself, then the regimen can be altered to make it more specific. Women presenting with a node under the arm, which is reported as containing cancer cells that are consistent with breast cancer, are treated as if they had breast cancer.

At autopsy for metastatic cancer presenting above the diaphragm as an unknown primary, the most common site of actual primary is lung cancer. If the presentation is below the diaphragm, pancreas is often found to be the primary site.

The outcome depends very much on the actual primary and should be individualised to each patient. A testicular cancer presenting as an unknown primary with metastatic disease could be cured, whereas if the actual primary was pancreatic cancer the course of the disease would be rapidly downhill.

SUMMARY

Cancer is more than 100 different diseases. We have illustrated the spectrum of cancers and their different behaviours, but have also demonstrated the principles of management that can apply to all, so that the behaviour of cancers not mentioned here can also be understood.

8

Prevention is better than cure

Martian sanitary science eliminated them years ago. A hundred diseases, all the fevers and contagions of human life, consumption, cancers, tumours and such morbidities, never enter the scheme of their life.

—*H.G. Wells,* War of the Worlds, *1897*

It should be our aim, like the Martians in *War of the Worlds*, to prevent disease rather than have to treat it. We should look forward to the day when prevention needs more than just one chapter in a book on cancer. In discussing the causes of cancer, we noted three simple things that prevent cancer. The first is to stop smoking tobacco. The second is to change our diets so that we eat more fresh fruit and vegetables and less fat. The third is to protect ourselves from prolonged exposure to the sun. We can add to that the opportunities that screening gives us, in cancer of the cervix, to treat precancerous conditions before they develop into cancer. Genetic screening gives us the chance to prevent cancer even if it means removing a healthy organ against the possibility that a cancer will develop in it. Finally, there are some drugs that are being trialled to prevent the development of cancer in people at risk.

STOP SMOKING

Leaving aside other major diseases, like airways disease and heart disease, ceasing to smoke will prevent the development of many lung cancers, mouth and throat cancers and bladder cancers. We would also expect to see reductions in kidney cancer and invasive prostate cancers. Stomach, pancreas and bowel cancers would be less frequent and even the incidence of lymphomas and leukaemias should decrease.

There must be several parts to a strategy to prevent smoking. Clever advertising that targets vulnerable groups such as adolescents must be limited. The power of advertising has been adequately demonstrated by the way the social customs of women have changed from non-smoking to smoking, with the subsequent impact on their death rate from lung cancer. At the same time as decreasing advertising, public education about the dangers of smoking must be increased. Non-smokers must be protected from the harmful effects of passive smoking by limiting smoking in enclosed spaces. Many offices and public transport vehicles in various parts of the world ban smoking. This is not necessarily because of enlightenment, but fear of litigation due to the harmful effects of passive smoking. Nonetheless, it has been an important step.

Education of individuals who give up smoking is important. Cutting down on the number of cigarettes smoked is not a good strategy. There is an addiction to nicotine which means that at times of stress the number of cigarettes is likely to climb again. Indeed, 'stress' is sometimes being caused by the nicotine withdrawal and responds to nicotine. Nor is changing to low-tar cigarettes very successful because it leads to longer and deeper inhaling to achieve the same fix. Also, the same cancer-causing chemicals are still being inhaled.

Patients should be encouraged to stop smoking right away rather than putting it off. They will need support, perhaps from a quit program, and may be helped by replacement nicotine as patches or gum. Negative perceptions about giving up should be countered. Weight gain, for example, is not mandatory unless

185

food is sought as solace for the lack of cigarettes. Positive benefits of giving up include having extra money for other pursuits. Even the old tale that there is no point to cancer patients giving up since it is like closing the stable door after the horse has bolted is incorrect. The chances of head and neck and lung cancer recurring may be decreased by stopping smoking.

Chewing tobacco, a habit of some sportsmen, is also dangerous because it exposes the lining of the mouth to cancer-causing agents. In India, tobacco and betel nut are often combined in the mouth and both can promote cancer.

PREVENTING CANCER WITH DIET

We have discussed diet and cancer in looking at the causes of cancer. It should be highlighted because it is a preventive strategy.

Fat

Strong associations have been found at an international level between the incidence of breast, colon, prostate and endometrial cancer and the intake per individual of fat. This, together with results from animal studies, led to the suggestion that fat should only provide 30 per cent of our energy. There are, however, many other factors, such as affluence, that could be associated with a country having a high fat intake. When case-control studies were done in breast cancer to look at this specifically, only a weak association was found and even this was not found in cohort studies. In animal studies, polyunsaturated fats were the culprits and it has even been suggested that mono-unsaturated fats are protective.

With large bowel cancer, any association seems to be with animal fat such as that found in red meat. This has been shown in case-controlled studies where there is also an association with total energy intake, that is, general overeating. This is coupled with the suggestion that a sedentary lifestyle may also be to blame.

The association reported in some case-controlled studies between fat and prostate cancer seems to be related to animal fats as well. There seems little association with vegetable fats.

A recommendation to people wanting to reduce their chance of developing cancer would be to limit their intake of animal fats through red meats. Also, they should not be over-weight and should exercise regularly.

Fibre

The association between fibre intake and cancer risk also needs further study. International studies comparing Africa with the West suggest increased dietary fibre is associated with decreased large bowel cancer, breast cancer and several other cancers including oesophageal, head and neck, stomach, prostate, endo-metrial and ovarian cancers. There are several difficulties with understanding this association.

First, fruit and vegetables may reduce your cancer risk but they contain other substances that may reduce cancer as well as fibre. Second, there are many different types of fibre and not all may be associated with decreased cancer risk. Bran cereal has been found to reduce the development of polyps in individuals with familial polyposis. Wheat bran is associated with decreased risk of bowel cancer in animals.

There may be a difference in the association between fibre and cancers at the top of the large bowel compared with those at the bottom. Large studies looking at bowel cancer risk and dietary fibre intake are still in progress. Dietary fibre appears to reduce the risk of breast cancer independently of fat intake. This may be secondary to the fact that fibre decreases production of some of the sex hormones but soy extracts can inhibit some of the signalling pathways in cancer cells.

In case-controlled studies the association with ovarian cancer is with vegetable fibres but not cereals. A vegetarian diet is also associated with a decreased risk of prostate cancer.

The recommendation for prevention at the current level of knowledge, therefore, would be to include a variety of different sources of fibre in the diet including fruits, vegetables and whole grains.

Vitamins and minerals

Vitamins and minerals also appear to have a part to play in preventing cancer. Part of the goodness of fruit and vegetables can be attributed to them, but it can be difficult to separate from other factors such as vegetable fibre. Specific studies have suggested a link between carotenoids and the prevention of smoking-related cancers, vitamin C and protection from stomach cancer, folate and cancer of the cervix, and calcium and large bowel cancer. Specific clinical trials to test these associations need to be very large and many are ongoing. Trials, to date, have shown mixed results. In lung cancer, for example, beta carotene and retinol have not been shown to reduce the incidence of lung cancer in smokers, but high-dose vitamin A has been shown to reduce the occurrence of second primaries after successful treatment of the first lung cancer.

There are certainly good reasonable theories about how vitamins and minerals could protect against cancer. They have been shown to block the action of cancer-causing chemicals. Vitamin A, beta carotene, vitamin C and selenium are antioxidants which can mop up cancer-causing agents. Vitamin A and derivatives, the retinoids, can slow growth and cause cells to differentiate—that is, to change to more mature forms. Finally, it is suggested that vitamins and minerals may affect the immune system but evidence for this is sparse and the subject of ongoing research.

A further difficulty with trials is that the process of developing cancer requires multiple steps over a long time and thus exposure to the dietary factor should be over a long time. It is also very difficult to judge what chemical action the nutrient has had and whether a step in the development of cancer has been blocked.

If vitamins and minerals are important to the body in the doses extracted from food, it does not follow that large doses as tablets or injections will have the same beneficial effects. They will certainly have different side effects. It would seem that the best preventive strategy at present is to eat foods containing the important vitamins and minerals. Although it may seem self-evident, vitamins and minerals used to prevent cancer may not be useful as a treatment for cancer, although much is written in the literature of alternative medicine advocating this. In fact, a developed cancer has progressed beyond the steps where these nutrients are thought to work, so you may be preventing the next cancer but not treating the established cancer.

A balanced diet

We have discussed what to eat to prevent cancer but there are some foods that may contain cancer-causing agents. Many plants contain natural pesticides as part of protecting themselves. Some have been found to inhibit and others to promote cancer, but the majority have not been tested. Without wishing to have this taken out of context by generations of small children, cabbage contains 49 natural pesticides, most of which have not been studied for cancer-causing potential or their ability to protect from cancer.

Sometimes it may be a contaminant of the food that is a problem. For example, aflatoxins produced by aspergillus can contaminate maize, corn and peanut crops. They have been particularly associated with liver cancer. Some countries have a regulatory program.

Some carcinogens can be introduced in the cooking of food. Heterocyclic aromatic amines (HAAs) are formed if foods, particularly meat, are exposed to high temperatures such as in frying, broiling or grilling but are not a problem with steaming, poaching, stewing or microwaving. The good old Aussie barbecue, with all its smoke, coats meat with polycyclic aromatic hydrocarbons, whereas cooking in an oven or microwave does not. The known carcinogenicity and the exposure, however, don't tell us what the actual risk to us is. This is particularly unclear because foods are also known to contain substances that work against these cancer-causing agents.

In summary, a diet designed to prevent cancer should have more fruit and vegetables and cereal and less red meat. This will provide fibre, vitamins and minerals and fewer animal fats. This does not mean cutting out food groups such as red meat altogether since we need some fat and iron and we don't want to create a diet that is deficient in other areas. Nor do we need to make life a misery by banning foods. We are talking about reaching a balance.

STAY OUT OF THE SUN

We have learned that short bursts of severe sun exposure can predispose to melanoma while more prolonged exposure causes non-melanoma skin cancers. The message of prevention is to keep covered by wearing hats and shirts and applying sunscreen. It should not, however, be thought that this practice allows safe prolonged sun exposure. It is far better to avoid sun exposure, particularly during the hottest part of the day.

Another aspect of cancer prevention is to protect the ozone layer in the atmosphere which screens out ultraviolet light. Reduction in the use of chlorofluorocarbons is one measure that will protect the ozone layer. It has been calculated that a 1 per cent decrease in ozone may cause a 2.7 per cent increase in non-melanoma skin cancer, so protection of the ozone layer is a sensible cancer prevention strategy.

DRUGS TO PREVENT CANCER

Chemopreventive drugs, or drugs to prevent cancer, suppress steps in the process of cancer development, which occurs over many years. Genetic changes can affect a whole area of cells. In head and neck cancer, for example, multiple cancers and second primary cancers occur in the squamous cell lining. There is a precancerous condition in the mouth where white plaques called leukoplakia are seen; although these can disappear, 30–40 per cent of them will progress to cancer if untreated.

Retinoids and carotenoids

The best studied chemopreventive agents are the relatives of vitamin A, the retinoids and the carotenoids. In leukoplakia a number of studies suggested benefit for both agents. Two randomised trials looked at beta carotene alone, and with retinol, and found significant reductions in leukoplakia over the no-treatment comparison. Five randomised studies of retinoids have provided valuable information. First, high doses for short periods have more side effects and the lesions recur quickly after stopping. Longer-term maintenance was more effective with retinoids as compared with beta carotene. Two trials of different retinoids given following treatment of head and neck cancer had different findings. One found that there was no difference in recurrence or survival but second cancers in the head and neck, oesophagus and lung were reduced. In the other trial no effect on second cancers was found. There are ongoing trials with retinoids and beta carotene in head and neck cancer.

Similarly, in lung cancer, trials of the use of retinoids to reduce the presence of abnormal cells in the lungs of heavy smokers yielded conflicting results. A randomised study showed no effect of the retinoids. Worse still, two trials of giving beta carotene to prevent lung cancer showed a greater rate of lung cancer in the treatment group, while a third study showed no difference. There are ongoing trials with retinoids as cancer prevention agents.

In other cancers, specific groups have been found to benefit. In breast cancer, postmenopausal women on a retinoid had a lower incidence of cancer occurring in the other breast and, incidentally, there was less ovarian cancer in the treated group. In the rare disorder, xeroderma pigmentosum, patients have a high incidence of skin cancers. These can be reduced by giving retinoids but this has not translated into usefulness in preventing

191

skin cancers in trials in the general population. Trials are ongoing to prevent other cancers such as cancer of the cervix, oesophagus, stomach, bladder lining and bowel. New retinoids and carotenoids with fewer side effects and different activity are currently being tested.

Aspirin

'Take two aspirin and see me in the morning' may be a cancer prevention strategy. Interest in aspirin and anti-inflammatory drugs is based on experiments in animals and two clinical observations. Patients taking these drugs for rheumatoid arthritis have a decreased incidence of cancer of the digestive tract. An anti-inflammatory drug causes shrinkage of the polyps in people with familial polyposis.

Six case-controlled studies and six of seven cohort studies showed a lower risk of colorectal cancer in people who take aspirin. One randomised blinded controlled study involving doctors showed no benefit in cancer prevention from taking aspirin for five years. The same study also looked at cardiovascular disease and the benefit in reduction in heart attacks in the doctors taking aspirin became so great that it was no longer appropriate to deprive one group of aspirin.

Why the difference between the randomised and case-controlled studies? It may be that people who choose to take aspirin look after their health better in general and eat better diets, so that the reduction in large bowel cancer is not due to the aspirin at all. It may also be that the duration of aspirin-taking in the controlled study was too short to prevent cancer, compared with longer durations in the epidemiological studies. Further studies will have to look at the duration and dose of aspirin, but it seems a promising preventive strategy for colorectal and maybe other cancers.

Hormones

There is no doubt that hormones given to patients can cause cancer. This was seen when oral contraceptives were given as a sequence of oestrogen followed by oestrogen with progesterone. This significantly increased the incidence of cancer of the endometrium (lining of the uterus). Changing to a combined preparation, which didn't use unopposed oestrogens (i.e. oestrogens alone), protected women on the pill against the risk of endometrial cancer. The combined oral contraceptive also reduced the risk of cancer of the ovary.

Hormone replacement therapy to provide relief for the symptoms of menopause also increased the risk of endometrial cancer when oestrogens were given unopposed. Again, prevention of this problem involved adding progestogens to the hormones given. Unopposed oestrogen will also increase the risk of breast cancer in this group but at the same time lowers the risk of cardiovascular disease, improving the overall death rate. Adding progestins could increase the chance of breast cancer and decrease the cardiovascular benefits, but this remains to be seen.

Tamoxifen given to postmenopausal women as additional therapy after the local treatment of breast cancer increases survival and decreases the incidence of second cancers in the opposite breast. A randomised trial was therefore commenced to assess the benefit of preventing breast cancer by using tamoxifen in healthy women at high risk of developing breast cancer. A trial of a drug with its own potential side effects in a healthy population is quite innovative and relies on the hope that the preventive effect on breast cancer is not counterbalanced by earlier side effects of the tamoxifen. Possible additional benefits of tamoxifen are its effects on lowering blood fats and reducing the loss of bone density seen in older women. The most worrying side effect is the increased incidence of endometrial cancer in the tamoxifen arm of the study. This illustrates why tamoxifen should not be used as a preventive agent until the results of the ongoing studies are known.

Trials of finasteride, a drug used in benign swelling of the prostate gland, are being conducted to see whether it will prevent prostate cancer. This is based on the drug's action in

193

inhibiting a chemical thought to be associated with the development of prostate cancer.

SUMMARY

We can prevent cancer by stopping cigarette smoking, avoiding sunburn and prolonged exposure to the sun and changing our diet to include less animal fat, particularly from red meat cooked at high temperatures or barbecued, and more fresh fruit and vegetables which contain fibre and the vitamins and minerals needed to prevent cancer. Trials of retinoids and carotenoids, aspirin and hormones such as tamoxifen may give us further strategies for preventing cancer.

9

Treating the symptoms

If the changes that we fear be thus irresistible, what
remains but to acquiesce with silence, as in the other
insurmountable distresses of humanity? It remains that
we retard what we cannot repel, that we palliate what
we cannot cure.

—Dictionary of the English Language, *Preface, Samuel Johnson*

Quality of life is a most important goal in treating patients with
cancer. We must control the symptoms caused by the cancer
so that individuals can continue with their lives. Curing a
tumour is the best way to eliminate the symptoms. Even partly
shrinking a tumour with chemotherapy or radiotherapy can be
very effective in relieving symptoms. We must balance the side
effects of the treatment with the beneficial effects.

Independent of anti-cancer treatments, there is much that
can be done to make patients comfortable. Palliative care is a
new specialty where symptom control has become the focus of
the expertise. Rather than involve palliative care doctors when
no further anti-cancer therapy can be given, we have adopted
a model of parallel care so that each specialty can contribute its
expertise throughout a patient's treatment. This ensures a holistic
approach. The topic of symptom control is the subject of whole

textbooks but it is important for us to see just how much can be done to relieve some of the common symptoms of cancer.

MANAGING PAIN

Pain is the symptom that most people fear when told they have cancer. Although probably 70 per cent of patients will experience chronic pain at some time during their illness, it is important to realise that cancers need not cause pain. In the liver, for example, the nerve endings are all in the capsule, or outer skin, of the liver and a cancer growing in its substance without stretching the liver will not cause pain. Similarly, cancers could grow in the lung without necessarily causing pain as a symptom.

The nature of cancer-related pain is that it is usually chronic or longstanding because that is the nature of the illness causing it. It is important to know that much can be done to relieve this symptom even when anti-cancer treatments have little more to offer.

There are different types of pain which require different treatments. For example, somatic pain is in skin or deeper tissues and is well localised, often described as dull or aching. Visceral pain is due to stretching pain fibres in organs in the abdomen or chest. It is often poorly localised and associated with sweating or nausea. Neuropathic pain can be due to cancer pressing on nerves or the spinal cord. It is often described as a burning pain with sudden shock-like sensations. Pain can be caused by the cancer or even the treatment. For example, if a nerve is damaged after surgery or radiotherapy, pain will result.

There are a few rules of thumb about taking pain medication for chronic cancer pain. The first is that the medication must be taken regularly so the concentration of the drug is maintained and the patient takes the next dose before the pain comes back. The second is that the dosage and type of medication is balanced against the pain. Fears of overdosing on opiate drugs like morphine, or becoming addicted to morphine, are unfounded.

If the dose is increased as the pain intensity increases, the drug will not have an overwhelmingly toxic effect. There is no upper limit to morphine's ability to control pain, irrespective of the dose, so a patient will never run out of pain relief and doesn't have to save morphine for a last resort. If the pain decreases, studies have shown that there is no problem in decreasing or stopping the drug.

Medication for cancer pain may start with simple pain-relieving drugs such as paracetamol. If this does not relieve the pain, combinations of paracetamol and codeine can be used. It is becoming more common, however, to use morphine much earlier for controlling chronic pain, particularly with the intro-duction of the long-acting morphines which are taken by mouth only once or twice each day. Short-acting morphine syrup can be taken to control pain that 'breaks through' the control of the long-acting tablet and its dose increased if regular additional doses of short-acting morphine are needed.

If patients are unable to swallow tablets, morphine can be given continuously under the skin through a small needle attached to a portable pump. Again, this allows continuous pain control. Further, small catheters can be placed next to the spinal cord where very low doses of opiates may relieve pain without as many side effects. Patches worn on the skin deliver the drug fentanyl and broaden the options for delivering pain medication.

Morphine can have side effects including drowsiness, nausea and constipation. These must be relieved and it is usual practice to begin a laxative at the same time as an opiate.

Depending on the type of pain, other drugs may be more effective than opiates and should be tried first or given in addition. Bone pain responds best to anti-inflammatory drugs such as aspirin. Bisphosphinates, which inhibit the cells that break down bone, are also useful and can prevent bone pain. Pain from the liver capsule can respond well to steroids such as prednisolone. Headache from raised pressure by cancer in the brain may also respond to steroids like dexamethasone. Neural-gic pain can respond to oral local anaesthetics such as mexiletine or anticonvulsants such as carbamazepine and even antidepressants.

The perception of pain is also important in the experience of pain and antidepressants, sedatives and drugs to reduce anxiety may need to be used with pain-relieving drugs to alleviate a patient's distress. Psychological counselling can also be helpful.

WEIGHT LOSS

Malnutrition with loss of appetite, weakness and wasting are thought to be associated with the cancer or with the body producing cytokines such as tumour necrosis factor or interleukin–1 which can change the breakdown of proteins, fats, sugars and starch. After an assessment of a patient's diet appropriate changes can be made. Sometimes these will be simple, such as replacing foods that cause discomfort with more palatable foods. Patients with liver involvement by cancer, for example, will often find that fatty foods and dairy products upset them but fruit and vegetables are more palatable. If the reason for not eating is mechanical, such as pressure on the stomach from cancer or fluid, small, more frequent meals may maintain an adequate intake. If nausea or vomiting due to cancer or its treatment is a problem, taking an anti-nausea tablet half an hour before eating will allow a better intake. Some people lose their sense of taste after chemotherapy. Increasing spicy flavours may make foods more palatable.

Dietary supplements in the form of drinks or powders may be useful for people who can't manage solid meals. More aggressive measures such as nourishment through a feeding tube into the stomach or even intravenously are only appropriate if the cancer is being actively treated or if survival is long enough to warrant feeding and there is a permanent problem with swallowing.

Eating is an important part of maintaining the quality of life. Even someone with an inoperable blockage of the bowel can still eat if a tube is placed through the skin into the stomach to vent any pressure built up by taking food by mouth into the stomach.

DIGESTIVE TRACT SYMPTOMS

We have discussed nausea and vomiting under the side effects of chemotherapy and there is a range of anti-nausea drugs and different routes of administration to use. It is most important to work· out the cause in a patient with cancer. Vomiting could be a symptom of cancer, particularly involving the brain, liver or stomach; it can be a side effect of treatment, due to a problem with the blood chemistry; or it can be due to other drugs such as opiates. They require different measures.

Constipation is a common problem. Sometimes it can be alleviated with a change in diet and patients should always be encouraged to drink plenty of fluids. Laxatives will often be required and enemas may be needed to relieve a longstanding problem. Care should be taken to rule out bowel obstruction due to cancer before any of these measures are tried.

Diarrhoea can be caused by irritation from a cancer, from the effects of chemotherapy or radiotherapy, or by an infectious agent. Most diarrhoea can be treated by stool-binding agents. One anomaly is spurious diarrhoea where the loose bowel motion is simply leakage past a bowel obstructed due to constipation.

BREATHING PROBLEMS

Shortness of breath can be a difficult symptom. If it is due to a cancer blocking a major airway, local radiotherapy or mechanical solutions such as lasers through a bronchoscope or stenting the airway open can be effective. If it is due to more widespread disease and no further anti-cancer treatments are available, steroids such as prednisolone can be helpful. Morphine to calm down the breathing can also increase the level of comfort.

EMERGENCY SYMPTOMS

There are several symptoms of cancer that need to be treated urgently to prevent serious problems. One of these that has already been mentioned is fever due to infection when the white blood cell count is low. Antibiotics should be administered as soon as possible to prevent the infection causing a dangerous fall in the blood pressure.

Another serious symptom is pain or, worse, weakness or numbness due to the pressure of a cancer on the spinal cord. This pressure must be relieved quickly with steroids, and then radiotherapy or surgery, to prevent loss of the use of arms or legs or bowel or bladder function. Swelling of the face and upper body from a cancer in the centre of the chest should also be promptly treated when the diagnosis is made.

Symptoms such as bleeding or blockage of bowel or bladder, or perforations of bowels, need to be treated on their merits, depending on their site and the type of cancer that has caused them. The non-specific effects of cancer—for example, elevations of blood calcium levels—are treated in the same way irrespective of the cause.

Patients often ask about the symptoms they are likely to have as their cancer becomes worse. You will see from the above examples that many different symptoms are possible, ranging from general symptoms like weight loss or tiredness to specific symptoms at the site of the cancer. The important fact is that there is a great deal that can be done to control the symptoms that a cancer will cause, quite apart from specific anti-cancer treatments.

PSYCHOSOCIAL SUPPORT

As part of multidisciplinary care, we provide clinical psychologists and social workers to support patients in adapting to their illness, but I am sure that the most important support comes from family and friends. Sometimes, problems arise because patients adapt quickly to their new situation with its new language and challenges, while friends and relatives may be less informed and unsure what to do. Patients tell me that sometimes they are abandoned by friends who can't cope with their illness.

Sometimes, the opposite happens and they are smothered with attention. I remember the old patient who was very angry because, once they found out he had cancer, his friends insisted on carrying his lawn bowls onto the green despite the fact that when he got out there he was still winning all the trophies. The message is that most patients want to get on with life and be treated as normal.

'Should we talk about it?' Most patients will want to discuss, at some time, their illness or the change to their life's plans with those closest to them. This can only occur if the parties aren't trying to protect each other by not discussing the cancer, or death, if they haven't got a curable cancer. Most doctors will try to give patients an accurate estimation of the time course of their illness because it is important for planning. I am suspicious of people who believe they have been given a specific number of weeks or months to live because it is not possible to be that accurate. I suspect that anything more than a ballpark figure—weeks to months, months to years—happens only in the movies.

The problem with cancer is not so much the reduced life expectancy as the uncertainty. It takes from people the ability to plan for the long term. Patients should be encouraged to prioritise the things they want to do and achieve a series of short-term goals. Planning for the worst and hoping for the best is a sensible strategy. It is important that all the people involved, including children (who reach an understanding at their own level), can be part of that planning.

Professional counselling may be required to provide patients with coping strategies for the abnormal situation in which they find themselves. Some may have specific problems such as an altered body image, or sexual and relationship problems that need to be worked through. Others, who have spent their life believing they are valued for what they do, may need to be counselled to see that they have value to those who love them for what they are, and being limited in what they can do does not signal the end of a valuable life.

SUMMARY

There are so many aspects to the quality of a life that it is little wonder we need a team approach to the treatment of cancer, particularly if maintaining a person's quality of life is our primary aim. I have shown in this chapter that there is much we can do to control the symptoms of cancer. We will continue to improve the outcomes of cancer treatment by research into its causes and management. We will continue to improve our care of patients if we continue to learn from them.

Glossary

ablation Remove (surgically) or destroy tissue.

adenocarcinoma Adeno refers to glands, that is groups of cells which secrete substances such as mucin. This is a cancer of gland-forming tissue, for example, the lining of the bowel. Under the microscope the cancer cells can be arranged in gland-like structures.

adenoma A benign tumour of gland-forming tissue. *See also* adenocarcinoma.

adjuvant therapy Treatment given in addition to the definitive local treatment of surgery or radiotherapy. An example is the use of hormone therapy or chemotherapy after surgery for breast cancer to prevent recurrence. The rationale is to treat patients at high risk of their disease returning. Although there is no visible disease when adjuvant therapy is given, it is designed to treat any microscopic disease which may remain.

aetiology The assigning of a cause.

aggressive When referring to cancers it means that the cancer is likely to grow or spread rapidly. Under a microscope, the aggressiveness of a cancer can be judged by the proportion of cells which are dividing.

alkylating agent Anti-cancer drug which binds chemically to the bases on DNA so that the cell cannot divide. Examples include nitrogen mustard, cyclophosphamide and melphalan.

amino acids   These are the building blocks of proteins. There are twenty and they each have a three-letter word in the genetic code so that a gene can act as the blueprint for a protein.

angiogenesis   The growth of new blood vessels. The development of an adequate blood supply is necessary for tumours to grow beyond 2 millimetres in size. Tumours can produce factors that stimulate the growth of these new vessels.

angiogram   A diagnostic imaging test where contrast is injected into blood vessels and x-rays taken. This can show the blood supply to organs or cancers.

antibody   Protein produced by the body's immune system as part of the defence against foreign organisms, such as the bacteria and viruses which cause infections. They interact with antigens on the surface of the invading organism.

antigen   A substance that when introduced into the body stimulates the production of antibodies.

antioxidant   A substance that prevents or delays the chemical reaction of oxidation. The formation of cancers may be prevented by antioxidants in the diet.

apoptosis   Programmed cell death. This is the process controlled by genes in which a cell will die when it has reached its life span. Alterations to genes can prevent this from happening in some cancers.

arthrogram   A diagnostic imaging test where contrast material is injected into a joint and x-rays taken to display the structures in the joint.

autocrine   Refers to a factor produced by a cell which acts upon that cell. The cell is self-regulating rather than being influenced by the cells around it.

biopsy   The examination of a piece of tissue taken from the body so that a diagnosis can be made. The term is often used for the procedure of removing the tissue.

basement membrane   Delicate membrane that underlies layers of cells and separates them from the surrounding tissue.

benign   Not cancerous. Usually a slow-growing group of cells that does not spread to distant sites.

cancer   An uncontrolled growth of cells invading the surrounding tissue, which has the ability to spread to distant sites through the bloodstream and lymphatic channels.

cadherin Protein on the cell surface involved in sticking the cells together.

carcinogen A cancer-producing factor or agent, such as chemicals, radiation and viruses.

carcinogenesis The process of development of a cancer. Usually involves a substance that can cause cancer (a carcinogen), such as a chemical, radiation or virus.

carcinoma A name given to cancers arising from cells which line body surfaces (called epithelial cells). These are to be distinguished from sarcomas which arise from supporting structures such as muscle or bone.

case-controlled study A study in which a group of people with cancer are matched with an identical group of patients without cancer and compared.

catheter A tube for passing into body canals. Most commonly refers to the tube passed into the bladder to drain urine.

chromosome Long strands of DNA in pairs contained in the nucleus or centre of cells. Each cell has 23 pairs of chromosomes which carry all the genetic information. They are divided into sections called genes.

clone The descendants produced by division from a single cell. The cells will all have the same genetic make-up unless mutation occurs.

cohort A specific group of people. In epidemiological studies a cohort study is performed by matching two groups of people for all characteristics except for the characteristic under study.

collagen Fibrous protein that forms the scaffolding between cells.

colonoscopy Examination of the inside of the large bowel using a long hollow flexible tube lit by optical fibres. The colonoscope is introduced into the bowel after the bowel contents have been cleared and can often be manipulated to see the length of the bowel. Biopsies can be taken of the lining of the bowel through the colonoscope.

colony Aggregate of cells.

colostomy An opening made surgically to drain the contents of the bowel out of the body through the wall of the abdomen. A collecting bag is worn over the hole or stoma. A colostomy may be temporary to allow for healing of the bowel after a surgical procedure or can be permanent if the extent of bowel removed or the position of the cancer does not allow the bowel to be connected to drain through the anus as it normally does.

compound A chemical consisting of two or more elements bound together in fixed proportions.

cytokine Substance produced by the body which enables one cell to affect the behaviour of another cell.

cytology The study of cells under the microscope. Cells are collected from body fluids such as sputum or the fluid which surrounds the spinal cord. Smears of the cervix yield cells. These cells can be examined for features that show they are cancer cells or exhibit precancerous changes.

cytoplasm The contents of a cell enclosed by the cell membrane, excluding the nucleus. It has the appearance of a transparent viscous fluid with various small structures included in it and is the site where all of the manufacturing and chemical processes take place.

debulking To remove the main mass of tumour (usually surgically). This may make it easier for other treatments to control what is left or may relieve symptoms.

differentiation The process where cells mature from a primitive stage to where they have a specialised function.

DNA Deoxyribonucleic acid, the chemical in the nucleus of each cell that stores all of the genetic information for the body and is the inherited material that determines an individual's characteristics. It consists of a string of nucleotides strung together. Each nucleotide has a sugar and one of four different bases: adenine (A), thymine (T), guanine (G) and cytosine (C). The bases are like an alphabet and the sequence of bases spells three-letter words. The strand of DNA is a spiral shape and two strands twist around each other in what is called a double helix. The bases on one spiral are always paired to the same base on the other spiral, A with T and C with G. To read the code the strands unravel.

dominant gene A gene which produces the characteristic it codes for even if it is passed on by only one parent.

embryo The name given to the new life developing in the uterus between conception and eight weeks.

emesis Vomiting. An anti-emetic drug is therefore one which prevents vomiting.

enzyme A protein that promotes the chemical reactions in the body without being used up during them. Many of the chemical reactions in the body are essential for producing energy and would not occur without the facilitation of the chemical reaction by enzymes. Enzymes can be targeted as one way of damaging cells.

epidemiology The study of the factors that affect the incidence of a disease. This is done by observing the variation in the incidence of disease under the differing conditions of life of different groups of people. Usually two large groups or populations of people are compared who are as similar as possible except for the characteristic being studied.

expressed When referring to a gene, this means that the product is made that the gene codes for.

extracellular matrix Structural tissue outside the cells which is often referred to as connective tissue and is the framework that holds the cells in place. It consists of proteins and sugars. To spread, tumours must penetrate this tissue.

extravasation Leakage of fluid out of a vessel. Usually applied to the leakage of drugs into the tissues surrounding a vein while they are being injected into the vein. With some drugs this can severely damage the surrounding tissues.

fibronectin One of the proteins that participate in the process of cancer cells binding to the basement membrane.

fractionate To divide into portions. In radiotherapy it refers to dividing the total dose into smaller doses and delivering them over a period of time, for example, five days a week for two weeks until the total desired dose is reached. This reduces the side effects of the therapy.

gene A length of DNA that contains enough information to code for making a protein. This may then determine an inherited characteristic.

hormone A chemical produced in one organ of the body that circulates by the bloodstream and exerts its effects on another organ in the body.

imaging Producing a representation of the form of an object. In relation to cancer may use x-rays or scans (such as CT scans) to create an image of the cancer.

isotope Different forms of a chemical element which vary by their weight. Some are radioactive and can be used for scanning organs which take them up.

laminin One of the proteins that help cancer cells to bind to the basement membrane.

lesion An area of damage or injury to an organ. It is usually circumscribed, such as an ulcer, a wound or a cancer.

lymphocyte A type of white blood cell that can make antibodies. It is part of the body's immune system and can migrate throughout the body. There are two main types, T-cells and B-cells. A virus attacking the T-cells is the cause of AIDS and results in infections and propensity to cancers, such as lymphomas and Kaposi's sarcomas.

malignant Cancerous. Has the ability to invade locally or spread to distant sites. Distinguished from a lump which is benign.

mammography Examination of the breasts using x-rays. The breast is compressed between two plates and can be x-rayed from above, from the side or obliquely.

mastectomy Surgical removal of the breast.

metastasis The spread of cancer away from its primary site (site of origin) to other parts of the body or secondary sites. A secondary cancer deposit in another organ is referred to as a metastasis. *See also* secondary.

micronutrient Food which the body must obtain from its environment to maintain health, though only needed in tiny amounts. Micronutrients are subdivided into vitamins, such as A, B, C, E, minerals such as calcium and selenium and non-nutrients such as flavonoids. In general they prevent damage to genes that cause cancer.

mitogen A substance that stimulates cell division.

molecule The smallest portion to which something can be divided without losing its chemical identity and ability to exist independently. Can be as little as one atom.

monoclonal antibody Antibodies of a particular type produced in the laboratory by selectively growing the cells which make the desired antibody.

motility Ability to move from one place to another.

mutation An alteration to the DNA of a cell which will be inherited by all of the daughter cells. Some mutations cause the loss of control over the growth of a cell which characterises cancer.

myelogram An x-ray designed to demonstrate the spinal cord by injecting contrast material into the spinal fluid which surrounds it.

neoplasm Literally a new growth. Refers to a cancer.

nitrosamine A cancer-causing chemical which can be formed in the body by the interaction of nitrates and nitrites with amines in food. Nitrates and nitrites can be added to food to preserve it (such as in cured meats). The high incidence of stomach and nasopharyngeal cancer in Asia may be due to the nitrosamine content of preserved food. The risk of nitrosamines can be reduced by eating fresh food.

nucleotide The building blocks of DNA. Consists of a sugar linked to a purine or pyrimidine base.

nucleus The part of the cell which contains the genetic material, DNA, in lengths called chromosomes. It is walled off by a membrane and is usually found near the centre of a cell.

oncogene Genes in the cell responsible for growth and multiplication which if switched on at the wrong time can cause uncontrolled growth, that is, cancer. Oncogenes can also be inserted into cells by viruses with the same outcome of loss of control of the cell's growth.

oncology The study of cancer. Now used to denote the medical specialty that involves the treatment of cancer, that is, radiation oncology, medical oncology, surgical oncology.

palliation Alleviation of the symptoms of a disease. Palliative care is the specialty which concentrates on controlling the symptoms of cancer.

pick-up rate The ability to detect a cancer when it is present.

population Group of people. Applying to a trial or study it is the group to be studied.

primary The original site where a cancer arose. The organ or tissue of origin.

prognosis Estimation in advance of the course of the disease. In cancer it is a forecast of the likely survival of the patient.

proliferation Reproduction and multiplication often causing a rapid increase in cell numbers.

promoter After initiation of the process of carcinogenesis many agents which often don't damage the genetic material can promote the development of the cancer. For example, they could stimulate proliferation or inhibit apoptosis.

prophylactic A measure taken to prevent disease or perhaps to prevent the side effects of a drug.

pseudopodia Temporary leg-like protrusion from the cell which helps to propel it.

receptor   A protein structure (often on the surface of cells) to which hormones and growth factors specifically bind (like inserting a key into a lock). Binding to the receptor triggers a series of signals necessary for the regulation of cell growth.

recessive gene   A gene coding for a characteristic where both copies of the gene, one from each parent must be inherited for the characteristic to become evident. This is compared to a dominant gene whose characteristic will be expressed irrespective of the gene inherited from the other parent. *See also* dominant gene.

regimen   The combination of drugs in a prescribed course of chemotherapy. There are some well-recognised combinations of drugs (drug regimens) that have been developed for specific cancers.

remission   The disappearance of all detectable cancer. This may not necessarily mean that the cancer has gone completely, since undetectable microscopic disease may remain which will eventually grow big enough to detect again. If, when the disease becomes undetectable, it has all gone then it will not return and the patient will be said to have been cured, but that is a retrospective assessment. The term partial remission is sometimes used to denote a 50 per cent or greater shrinkage of a cancer.

retinoid   A relative of vitamin A which can prevent the development and growth of some cancers.

sarcoma   A cancer arising from the connective tissues such as bone or muscle. To be distinguished from a carcinoma which arises from cells lining body surfaces.

secondary   The distant site to which a primary cancer spreads. The term used to describe the cancer at that site which is also called a metastasis. The cancer looks like the primary and is treated according to its primary site. *See also* metastasis.

sigmoidoscopy   Examination of the interior of the lower end of the large bowel, the sigmoid colon, with a flexible or rigid tube with a light.

signal transduction   Refers to the process of transmitting a message from outside a cell to the genetic material in the nucleus. The transfer of the signal is initiated by a hormone or growth factor binding to a receptor on the surface of the cell and a series of biochemical events occur to transfer the message to the nucleus.

somatic cell   A cell of the body. Unlike a germ cell (ovum or sperm), if there are any changes to the genetic material in a somatic cell the changes will not be passed on to the next generation.

spindle A fusiform structure. At the time of cell division when the genetic material has to be separated into two daughter cells, the chromosomes line up along protein fibres which run from one end of the cell to the other. The contraction of this protein spindle draws the chromosomes apart.

staging Determining the extent of cancer by imaging the body to see how far it has spread. The stage of a cancer can be associated with its prognosis and can determine whether it can be adequately treated with local treatments such as surgery or radiotherapy.

stem cell A group of cells in any tissue, such as bone marrow or bowel lining, that is capable of new growth. When stem cells divide one of the cells differentiates and matures while the other remains as a stem cell. Stem cells remain a source of new cells. Stem cells in the bone marrow are the source for replacement of circulating blood cells. The stem cells can be stimulated to migrate into the blood to be collected and can be used instead of harvesting bone marrow to replenish the bone marrow after high doses of chemotherapy.

stent A device for keeping a tube patent. For example, in the lung a stent may be inserted through a bronchoscope and springs open to keep the airway walls from being compressed by a cancer.

tissue A region consisting mainly of cells of the same type bound together by the material between them.

tomograph A radiographic cut through the body. This can be achieved by rotating the x-ray around a fixed point so that all except the area being studied is blurred. CT scans take cross-sectional images by taking multiple small images that are built into a picture by a computer.

trace element A substance usually part of the diet that must be available to the body for its health but is only required in small amounts. Iodine for thyroid function would be one example. Trace elements may be part of hormones or enzymes.

trauma Injury or wound.

tumour A lump or swelling. This can refer to either benign or cancerous lumps.

vitamin Substance which takes part in essential chemical processes in the body cannot be made by the body so must be included in the diet. Deficiencies of the fat-soluble vitamins A and E may be associated with the development of cancer, since vitamin A is essential for normal cell growth and vitamin E can help prevent the conversion of nitrates and nitrites to cancer-causing nitrosamines.

virus The smallest forms of life consisting of genetic material which can copy itself only by invading a cell and using the cell's mechanisms for replicating genetic material.

Reading list

DeVita V.T. Jr, Hellman S., Rosenberg S.A. eds. *Cancer Principles and Practice of Oncology*, 5th edn. Philadelphia: Lippincott–Raven, 1997.

Macdonald J.S., Haller D.G., Mayer R.J. eds. *Manual of Oncologic Therapeutics*, 3rd edn. Philadelphia: J.B. Lippincott, 1995.

Peckham M., Pinedo H., Veronesi U. eds. *Oxford Textbook of Oncology*. Oxford: Oxford University Press, 1995.

South Australian Health Commission. *Epidemiology of Cancer in South Australia 1977 to 1996*. Adelaide: South Australian Cancer Registry, 1997.

Additional references

Bradley T.R., Metcalf D. The growth of mouse bone marrow cells in vitro. *Australian Journal of Experimental Biology and Medical Science* 1966, 44: 287–294.

Burkitt D.P. Epidemiology of cancer of the colon and rectum. *Cancer* 1971, 28: 3–13.

Coley W.B. A report of recent cases of inoperable sarcoma successfully treated with mixed toxins of erysipelas and Bacillus prodigiosus. *Surgical Gynaecology and Obstetrics* 1911, 13: 174.

Feinstein A.R., Sosin D.M., Wells C.K. The Will Rogers phenomenon. Stage migration and new diagnostic techniques as a source of misleading statistics for survival in cancer. *New England Journal of Medicine* 1985, 312(25): 1604–1608.

Friedman L.S., Ostermeyer E.A., Lynch E.D., Szabo C.I., Anderson L.A., Dowd P., Lee M.K., Rowell S.E., Boyd J., King M.-C. The search for BRCA1. *Cancer Research* 1994, 54(24): 6374–6382.

Goodman L.S. et al. Nitrogen mustard therapy: use of methyl-bis (beta-chlorethyl) amine hydrochloride and tris (beta-chlorethyl) amine hydrochloride for Hodgkin's disease, lymphosarcoma, leukaemia and certain allied and miscellaneous disorders. *Journal of the American Medical Association* 1946, 132: 126–132.

Harris R., Leininger L. Clinical strategies for breast cancer screening: Weighing and using the evidence. *Annals of Internal Medicine* 1995, 122: 539–547.

Li F.P., Fraumeni J.F. Soft tissue sarcoma, breast cancer and other neoplasms. A familial syndrome? *Annals of Internal Medicine* 1969, 71: 747–752.

Olver I.N., Aisner J., Hament A., Buchanan L., Bishop J.F., Kaplan R.S. A prospective study of topical Dimethyl sulphoxide (DMSO) for treating anthracycline extravasations. *Journal of Clinical Oncology* 1988, 6: 1732–1735.

Rosenberg B., Van Camp I., Krigas T. Inhibition of cell division in Escherichia coli by electrolysis products from a platinum electrode. *Nature* 1965, 205: 698.

Rosenberg S. Principles of cancer management: surgical oncology. In DeVita, V.T. Jr, Hellman S., Rosenberg S.A. *Cancer Principles and Practice of Oncology*, 5th edn. Philadelphia: Lippincott–Raven, 1997, p. 295.

Southern E. Detection of specific sequences among DNA fragments separated by gel electrophoresis. *Journal of Molecular Biology* 1975, 98: 503–517.

Spiegel D., Bloom J.R., Kraemer H.C., Gottheil E. Effect of psychological treatment on survival of patients with metastatic breast cancer. *Lancet* 1989, ii: 888–891.

Useful Websites for information on cancer

National Cancer Institute USA http://www.nci.nih.gov
CancerNet http://wwwicic.nci.nih.gov/
Oncolink http://cancer.med.upenn.edu/
Medicine on Line http://wwwmeds.com/mol/welcome.html
Cancerhelp UK http://medweb.bhan.ac.uk/cancerhelp/
International Union Against Cancer http://www.uicc.ch/
Australian Cancer Network http://ludwig.edu.au/ACN/acs.html
National Breast Cancer Centre http://www.nbcc.org.au

Index

acquired immunodeficiency
  syndrome, 46, 141, 151–52, 176,
  180
actinomycin, D, 107
adenoma, 81
adjuvant,
  chemotherapy, 124, 160, 165, 173
  hormone, 128
  immunotherapy, 174
  radiotherapy, 156, 161, 165
adrenal gland, 129
  cancer, 109, 180
aflatoxin, 40, 189
AIDS *see* acquired immunodeficiency
  syndrome
airways disease, 33, 185
alcohol, 34, 119, 146, 148, 156, 163
Alexander, Colonel S.F., 105
alkylating agent, 48, 105, 106, 107,
  115, 123, 124, 127
allergy, 117
amino acid, 4
amsacrine, 107
anaemia, 121, 160, 179
anal cancer, 162
analine dye, 37, 145
angiogenesis, 17
  anti-angiogenesis factor, 136
angiogram, 63, 66
angiosarcoma, 37
anthracycline, 114, 116, 122, 123,
  126, 166, 177

antibiotics, 120, 200
  antitumour, 106, 107
antibody, 13, 19, 56, 130, 131
  monoclonal, 134
antigen, 13, 56, 71, 130, 131, 132,
  133, 134
antimetabolites, 106, 107, 115
antioxidant, 40, 188
antisense, 136
anxiety, 77, 198
apoptosis, 11, 96, 115
arsenic, 37
arthrogram, 63
asbestos, 21, 32, 35, 36, 180
  chrysotile, 36
  crocidolite, 36
asparaginase, 107, 108
aspirin, 49, 192, 194, 197
atomic bomb, 43, 152
Australia
  Aborigine, 45
  incidence, 139–40, 150
  melanoma, 85
  mesothelioma experience, 36
  mortality, 139–40

B symptoms, 175
bacillus Calmette-Guerin, 131, 173
bacteria, 47, 106, 108, 109, 110,
  119, 120, 148
  Escherichia coli, 110
  helicobacter pylori, 47, 149

217

barium
  enema, 82
  swallow, 159
Baruch, Bernard, 89
base, 4, 5, 57
basement membrane, 14, 15, 16
BCG *see* bacillus Calmette-Guerin
Beatson, George, 128
Becquerel, Antonie, 95
benign, 2, 53, 146
benzene, 37, 152
betel nut, 186
bias, 21, 80, 113, 143
  lead time, 74
biological therapy, 90, 130, 136
biopsy, 51, 52, 53, 54, 56, 72, 73,
  132
bisphosphonate, 167, 179, 197
bladder, 117, 123, 200
bladder cancer, 33, 37, 41, 85, 98,
  108, 125, 144, 173, 184
  squamous cell, 47, 145
  superficial, 93, 132, 192
  transitional cell, 145, 173
blast crisis, 178
bleomycin, 106, 107, 118, 119, 171,
  175
blinding, 21
blood, 13, 52, 59, 60, 160, 177,
  178, 182, 199
  bloodstream, 14, 15, 16, 19, 104,
    111, 156, 170
  vessels, 17, 136
bone cancer, 27, 101
bone marrow, 60, 127, 172, 176,
  177, 179
  stem cells, 120, 127
  suppression, 117, 119, 120, 127
  bowel cancer, 12, 27, 30, 38, 39,
    49, 77, 81, 87–8, 91, 93, 94,
    98, 111, 139, 140, 142, 147,
    160–2, 185, 186, 187, 188, 192
Bradley, T.R., 120
brain tumour, 27, 111, 154, 155, 181
breast cancer, 14, 27, 28–30, 31, 32,
  35, 38, 39, 40, 44, 48, 50, 55,
  78–9, 80, 86–7, 90–92, 94, 98,
  99, 101, 111, 125, 128, 129, 139,
  140, 141, 146–7, 164, 169, 179,
  182, 186, 187, 191, 193

bronchoscopy, 158, 199
bryostatins, 110
Bugula neitina, 110
Burkitt, D.P., 12, 39
  lymphoma, 12, 47
busulphan, 107, 178

CA-125, 85
cadherin, 15
calcium, 19, 158, 179, 188, 200
Camptotheca acuminata, 110
camptothecan analogues, 162
cancer *see specific types*
carbamazepine, 197
carboplatin, 107, 109
carcinogenesis, 9, 24, 30
  carcinogen, 33, 39, 40, 189
Caribbean, 110
carmustine, 107
case control study, 21, 80, 82, 85,
  142–3, 186, 192
cell, 3, 5, 8, 9, 10, 13, 14, 22, 52,
  135
  blood, 13
  clone, 115
  cycle, 6, 7, 8, 11, 107, 127
  division, 6, 7, 8, 9, 11, 23
  germ, 25
  line, 111
  somatic, 23, 27, 30
  stem, 6
  tumour, 15, 16, 17, 20
cervical cancer, 46, 48, 80–1, 102,
  141, 145, 167, 184, 188, 192
cervical intraepithelial neoplasia, 80
chemoprevention, 190
chemotherapy *see specific drugs*
Chernobyl, 101
childhood cancer, 124, 181
  leukaemia, 125
  sarcoma, 125
  Wilm's tumour, 125
chlorambucil, 107, 121, 176, 178
chlorination, 41
cholesterol, 37, 148
choriocarcinoma, 125
chromosome, 4, 5, 8, 27, 29, 36,
  56, 58, 178
  Philadelphia, 178
cigarette *see* tobacco smoking

CIN *see* cervical intraepithelial neoplasia
cisplatin, 107, 108–9, 118, 119, 122, 123, 126, 156, 157, 158, 160, 167, 168, 171, 173
Clowes, George, 104
clubbing, 158
coal, 42
codeine, 197
coffee, 145
cohort, 21, 141, 143, 192
colchicine, 105
Coley, William, 131
collagen, 15
colonoscopy, 77, 82, 83, 88, 161
colostomy, 94, 161, 163
constipation, 158, 160, 197, 199
contrast media, 63, 64, 67
    barium, 63
    gastrograffin, 63
control group, 21, 143
corticosteroid, 155, 200
    dexamethasone, 155, 197
    prednisolone, 175, 176, 178, 179, 197, 199
cough, 156, 158
CT scan *see* scan
Curie, Marie, 95
cyclophosphamide, 107, 118, 121, 122, 123, 145, 166, 167, 176
cystoscope, 93, 173
cytokine, 131, 134, 198
    IL-2, 131, 132, 133
    interleukin, 131, 132
    interleukin, 1, 198
    tumour necrosis factor, 198
cytology, 52
cytoplasm, 3, 5, 96
cytosine arabinoside, 107, 110, 177
cytotoxic drugs *see specific drugs*

dacarbazine, 107, 118, 174, 175
daunorubicin, 107
deoxyribonucleic acid, 3, 5, 8, 9, 10, 18, 23–4, 30, 31, 40, 42, 43, 45, 47, 55, 56–7, 58–9, 73, 96, 105–7, 108, 109, 115, 127, 135
depression, 77
diarrhoea, 160, 199
didemnin B, 110
diet, 33, 37–8, 141, 142, 144, 145, 146, 147, 148, 149, 151, 184, 186, 187, 188, 189, 194, 198
    vegetarian, 187
digital rectal examination, 84
DMSO, 117
DNA *see* deoxyribonucleic acid
docetaxel, 107
doxorubicin, 106, 107, 118, 121, 166, 168, 173, 175, 176, 179, 180
DRE *see* digital rectal examination
dysplastic naevus syndrome, 85

Ehrlich, Paul, 104
electromagnetic fields, 41, 42, 152
electron microscope, 59
emesis *see* vomiting
endometrial cancer, 48, 129, 168, 186, 187, 193
endoscope, 52, 92, 156, 159
enema, 62, 199
environment, 24, 30, 31–3, 35, 37, 42, 50, 114, 142, 148, 152
enzyme, 15, 16, 57
epidemiology, 32, 137, 141, 142–4, 145, 146, 147, 149, 151, 152, 153, 164, 192
epipodophyllotoxins, 114
epirubicin, 107, 160
etoposide, 107, 157, 171
exercise, 146, 148, 186
extracellular matrix, 15, 16, 17
extravasation, 116–17

faecal occult blood test, 81, 82, 88
familial polyposis coli, 27, 91, 187
fat, 38–9, 142, 144, 148, 184, 186, 193, 198
    animal, 148, 186, 190, 194
    mono-unsaturated, 39, 186
    polyunsaturated, 39, 186
    saturated, 39
    vegetable, 187
Feinstein, A.R., 72
α fetoprotein *see* marker
fever, 175, 178, 200
Fibonacci series, 112
fibre, 39, 142, 148–9, 186–7, 190, 194
fibronectin, 15, 16
finasteride, 193
flow cytometer, 56, 57

fludarabine phosphate, 107, 178
5 fluorouracil, 106, 107, 115, 121,
    122, 127–8, 156, 160, 161, 162,
    163, 166
foetus, 117, 123
Fraumeni, Joseph, 27

gadolinium, 67
gamma globulins, 178
gamma ray, 70, 71, 95
gemcitabine, 158
gene, 5, 6, 9, 14, 18, 23, 27, 33,
    37, 47, 57, 13
  amplification, 10
  APC, 27
  BRCA 1, 29, 30, 86, 87
  BRCA 2, 29, 30
  carrier, 25, 26
  dominant, 24, 25, 26, 27
  expression, 6, 7
  genetic counselling, 87
  human genome project, 37
  multidrug resistance gene, 115
  oncogene, 9, 10, 22, 43, 111
  proto-oncogene, 9, 10, 11
  p53, 27, 28, 29, 115
  recessive, 25, 26
  regulation, 10
  smoking, 147
  therapy, 18, 90, 135, 136
  tumour suppressor gene, 10, 11,
    22, 27, 28, 43, 86, 135
Gilman, 105
glandular fever, 47
Goodman, L.S., 105
growth factor, 7, 9, 10, 19, 108,
    111, 120, 127, 132, 135, 177
  G-CSF, 120, 177
growth fraction, 11
Grubbe, E.H., 95

hair, 117, 121
Halsted, William, 90
βHCG *see* markers
head and neck cancer, 33, 34, 98,
    108, 125, 156, 182, 184, 187,
    190, 191
  nasal sinus cancer, 37
  nasopharyngeal cancer, 40
  squamous cell, 156

heart disease, 33, 37, 101, 185, 192,
    193
  pumping power, 122
herbicide, 41
  2,4 D, 41
heterocyclic aromatic amines (HAA),
    189
hexamethylmelamine, 107
Hippocrates, 3
Hiroshima, 43, 152
Hodgkin, Thomas, 150
Hodgkin's disease, 92, 105, 125,
    128, 141, 150, 175
homosexual, 152
hormone, 7, 19, 31, 32, 40, 47, 49,
    93, 101, 128, 136, 146, 147, 156,
    158, 165–6, 169, 170, 180, 192,
    194
  androgen, 128, 129, 130
  anti-androgen, 130
    flutamide, 130
  aromatase inhibitors, 129
    aminoglutethimide, 129
  female, 164
  gonadotrophin releasing hormone,
    129
  luteinising hormone releasing
    hormone, 169
  male, 144
    testosterone, 169
  oestrogen, 128
    receptor (ER), 128, 129, 165
  oral contraceptive, 48, 146, 192
  parathyroid, 19
  progestogen, 129, 193
    medroxyprogesterone acetate,
    129, 168
    receptor, 165
  receptor, 165, 166
  replacement therapy, 48, 146, 193
  sex, 144, 187
hybridisation, *in situ*, 58
  fluorescent *in situ* hybridisation, 58
hydrocarbons, 41
hydroxyurea, 107, 178
hysterectomy, 167

idarubicin, 107
ifosfamide, 107, 123, 179
imaging, 60
immune system, 13, 19, 45, 49, 56,

INDEX

90, 130–1, 132, 133, 134, 141, 151, 188
immunoglobulin, 178
immunohistochemistry, 55–6
immunosupression, 152, 180
immunotherapy, 90, 131, 136, 174
impotence, 168
incidence, 139, 141, 142, 143, 145, 152
incontinence, 168, 169
infection, 45, 46, 47, 120, 121, 138, 142, 177, 178, 179, 200
  pneumocystis, 152
  secondary, 121
    thrush, 1, 21
infertility, 117, 123
inflammation, 54
inheritance, 23, 24, 25, 28, 29, 30, 33, 50, 148
interferon, 133–4, 174, 178
iodine, 103, 180
irinotecan, 107, 110
isotope, 71, 96, 103, 134, 170
  strontium, 170

Kaposi, Moritz, 152
Kaposi's sarcoma, 46, 141, 152, 180
kidney, 19, 117, 122, 123, 179
kidney cancer, 33, 94, 111, 125, 131, 134, 172, 181, 185
  nephroblastoma, 181
  Wilm's, 181
King, Mary-Claire, 29

laminin, 15, 16
laparoscope, 52
laparotomy, staging, 92
laser, 102, 158, 159, 199
Lee, Rose, 95
leucoplakia, 191
leucovorin, 161, 162
leukaemia, 27, 33, 37, 41, 43, 44, 49, 52, 101, 105, 110, 111, 124, 127, 151–2, 154, 174, 176, 177, 185
  acute lymphoblastic, 181
  acute myeloid, 177–8, 181
  childhood, 125, 151, 181
  chronic, 125, 133, 177
  chronic lymphatic, 178
  chronic myeloid, 177

lymphatic, 177
  T-cell, 152
Li, Frederick, 27
Li–Fraumeni syndrome, 27–8
linear accelerator, 95, 102
liposome, 180
liver cancer, 14, 35, 40, 46–7, 163, 189
lomustine, 107, 155
lung cancer, 32–4, 36, 37, 41, 85, 98, 108, 111, 139, 141, 156, 182, 185, 188, 191
  non-small cell, 125, 156, 158, 171
  small cell, 125, 156
lymph glands, 14, 54, 55, 56, 61, 65, 92, 98, 156, 157, 158, 164–5, 166, 171, 173, 174, 175, 176, 178, 182
lymphatic channels, 14
lymphocyte, 13, 130, 131, 134
  T-lymphocyte, 132
  tumour infiltrating, 135
lymphogram, 61, 66
lymphoma, 41, 46, 47, 49, 54, 56, 98, 101, 105, 111, 124, 125, 127, 133, 141, 150, 151–2, 154, 174–5, 185
  Burkitt's, 151
  high grade, 176
  intermediate grade, 176
  low grade, 125, 176, 178

malaria, 47
mammogram, 44, 62, 63, 77, 78–9, 87, 182
mandrake, 107, 110
marker, 60, 165, 172, 182
  CA-125, 167
  carcinoembryonic antigen (CEA), 161
  α fetoprotein, 60, 170
  β human chorionic gonadotrophin (HCG), 60, 170, 171
  prostate specific antigen (PSA), 170
mastectomy, 87, 90, 93, 164
meat, 39, 186, 187, 189, 190, 194
melanin, 45
melanoma see skin cancer
melphalan, 107, 179
menopause, 48, 146, 165, 168, 193

221

mercaptopurine, 107
mesna, 123
mesothelioma, 32, 35, 36, 180
meta-analysis, 165
metastasis, 13, 14, 18, 19, 93, 104,
    124, 158, 161, 166, 170, 174,
    179, 182
Metcalf, D., 120
methotrexate, 106, 107, 115, 121,
    123, 166, 173
mexiletine, 197
micronutrients, 40
microtubules, 106
minerals, 188–9, 190, 194
mitogen, 7
mitomycin, 107, 163
mitosis, 7, 8
mitotane, 107, 109
mitoxantrone, 107
morphine, 196, 197, 199
mortality, 139, 143, 145, 152
motility, 16, 140, 141
MRI scan see scan
mutation, 9, 10, 11, 22–3, 24, 25,
    27, 28, 30, 33, 41, 48, 50, 74,
    86, 91
myelogram, 61, 63
myeloma, 60, 125, 154, 179

Nagasaki, 43, 152
nausea, 117, 118–9, 155, 196, 197,
    198, 199
navelbine, 158
nerve, 19
    damage, 117, 123
neutrons, 103
nitrogen mustard, 105, 106, 107,
    118, 175
nitrosamine, 40, 149, 159
Northern blot, 57
nuclear medicine, 61, 69, 73
nucleus, 3, 5, 22, 96, 128
nystatin, 121

obesity, 48, 146
oedema, cerebral, 155
oesophageal cancer, 98, 159, 187,
    191, 192
oestrogen, 32, 40, 48, 193
oncology, 3
ondansetron, 119

ovarian cancer, 30, 48, 85, 87, 93,
    108, 111, 167, 181, 182, 187,
    191, 193
ovary, 128, 129
ozone layer, 45, 150, 190
    chlorofluorocarbons, 190

paclitaxel, 107, 117, 121, 167
pain, 155, 158, 160, 170, 172, 175,
    196, 197, 198, 200
    neuropathic, 196, 197
    somatic, 196
    visceral, 196
pancreatic cancer, 33, 163, 182, 185
Pap smear, 46, 52, 80, 141
Papanicolaou, George, 80
paracetamol, 197
paraneoplastic syndrome, 19
parasites, 47, 145
    schistosoma haemotobium, 47, 145
pathologist, 51, 53, 55, 56, 59, 160,
    165
Pavlov, 118
percutaneous endoscopic gastrostomy,
    159
periwinkle, 106, 109, 110
pesticides, 41, 189
PET scan see scan
photons, 103
pituitary gland, 128, 129
platelet, 119, 120
Podophyllin peltatum, 110
podophyllotoxins, 107, 110
pollutant, 32, 41, 42
polycyclic aromatic hydrocarbons, 189
polymerase chain reaction, 58
polyp, 27, 30, 33, 52, 161, 187, 192
Pott, Percival, 35
powerlines, 41, 42
prednisolone see corticosteroids
pregnancy, 123, 145, 146, 152
probe, 57–8
procarbazine, 107, 108, 155, 175
prostate cancer, 30, 31, 39, 77,
    83–4, 88, 94, 125, 129, 139, 140,
    141, 144, 168, 170, 182, 185,
    186, 187, 193–4
prostate specific antigen (PSA) see
    markers
protein, 4, 8, 9, 10, 13, 15, 18, 57,
    60, 73, 108, 198

Bence Jones, 60, 179
p-glycoprotein, 115
structural, 15
tumour specific, 133
PSA *see* prostate specific antigen
pseudopodia, 15
psychologist, 200
pump, portable infusion, 127, 162, 197

radiation, 9, 23, 42, 43, 69, 77, 96, 101, 147, 151
acute effects, 100, 102
field, 97, 100, 102
inverted Y, 175
mantle, 175
ionising, 42, 43, 96
late effects, 100
monoclonal antibody, 134
radium, 43, 95
reaction, 99
seeds, 169
tolerance to, 100
ultraviolet, 43, 45, 190
uranium, 43, 95
radiologist, 60
radiotherapy, 27, 44, 66, 89, 90, 92, 93, 94, 95–104, 124, 136, 147, 155, 156, 157–8, 159, 160, 163, 164, 167, 168, 169, 170, 171, 173, 174, 175, 176, 179, 180, 181, 182, 195, 199, 200
chemotherapy combination, 126
fraction, 97, 102
half-body, 98, 170
hyperfractionation, 97
stereotactic radiosurgery, 103, 155
total-body, 98
radon, 42, 43, 147, 152
receptor, 7, 15, 16
registry, cancer, 138–9, 153
hospital, 138–9
population, 138–9
resistance, 114–16
genetic, 114
sanctuary sites, 114
retinoblastoma, 25, 27
rheumatoid arthritis, 151, 192
ribonucleic acid, 4, 5, 6, 8, 10, 57, 58, 73, 106, 136, 162
RNA *see* ribonucleic acid

Roentgen, Wilhelm, 62, 95
Rogers, Will, 72, 114
Rosenberg, Barnett, 108

sarcoma, 3, 27, 93, 125, 179, 181
scan, 51, 60, 61
bone, 61, 70
computerised tomography (CT) scan, 44, 61, 64–6, 67, 71, 72, 73, 92, 97, 103, 155, 156, 182
SPECT, 71
magnetic resonance imaging (MRI), 61, 66–7, 71, 73, 155
magnetic resonance spectroscopy, 67
positron emission tomography (PET), 61, 67, 71
screening, 60, 62, 74–87, 90, 138, 141, 160, 164, 184
genetic, 86, 88, 184
scrotal cancer, 35
secondary cancer, 13, 15, 16, 17, 54, 55, 56, 59, 72, 94, 174
seizure, 155
serotonin receptor antagonist, 119
sigmoidoscopy, 82, 83
signal transduction, 7, 11
simulator, 102
skin cancer, 37, 44, 45, 84, 98, 173, 191–2
melanoma, 45, 55, 84–5, 88, 92, 111, 125, 131, 132, 133, 134, 135, 140, 149
non-melanoma, 45, 149, 150, 173–4, 190
Smith, Edwin, 90
smoking *see* tobacco smoking
Southern blot hybridisation, 57
sperm, 6, 123
Spiegel, D., 50
spindle, 7, 107
stent, 199
stomach cancer, 23, 47, 85, 141, 149, 160, 185, 187, 188, 192
stress, 49, 50, 142, 185
sulphur mustard, 105
sun exposure, 37, 45, 84, 150, 184, 190, 194
surgery, 89, 90–5, 124, 136, 155, 156, 157, 159, 160, 161, 162,

163, 164, 167, 168, 169, 171,
172, 174, 179, 180, 181, 196, 200
sweats, 175, 196

tamoxifen, 128, 129, 166, 168, 193,
194
taste, 198
taxane, 114, 158, 166
Taxus brevifolia, 110
TB, 131
technetium, 70
teniposide, 107
testicular cancer, 60, 85, 108, 124,
125, 141, 168, 170–2, 182
non-seminomatous, 171
Tetha crypta, 110
thioguanine, 107
thiotepa, 107
thyroid cancers, 93, 101, 180
tobacco smoking, 31, 32, 33, 36, 37,
41, 42, 49, 50, 140, 142, 144,
145, 147, 151, 156, 159, 184,
185, 186, 188, 191, 194
passive, 33, 143, 147, 185
topotecan, 107, 110
trace elements, 38, 40
selenium, 149, 188
tracheostomy, 156
transplant, 94
bone marrow, 95, 166, 176–7,
178, 179
liver, 94, 163
organ, 94, 151
stem cell, 127, 166, 176
trauma, 12, 13
trials, 1, 12, 20, 21, 73, 82, 84–5,
111–13, 130, 136, 141, 142, 159,
161, 162, 164, 165, 166, 169,
179, 180, 184, 188, 191, 192, 193
Trididemnum solidum, 110
tumour doubling, 11, 12

ulcer, 117
mouth, 121
ultrasound, 61, 67–9, 72
Doppler, 69
transrectal (TRUS), 84
United States
bowel cancer, 147–8
incidence, 140
mortality, 140

National Cancer Institute, 50, 111
prostate cancer, 144
unknown primary cancer, 181–2
uterine cancer, 167

vaccine,
pneumococcal, 178
tumour, 132–3, 174
vaginal cancer, 48
venous access device, 117
vinblastine, 106, 107, 121, 173, 175
vinca alkaloids, 109, 110, 114, 123
vinca rosea Linn, 110
vincristine, 106, 107, 118, 155, 175,
176
vindesine, 107
vinyl chloride, 36
virus, 9, 10, 11, 23, 31, 46, 59, 133,
135
Ebstein-Barr virus, 47, 150–1
hepatitis B virus, 47, 163
HTLV 1, 152
human immunodeficiency virus
(HIV), 46, 152
papilloma, 46, 80, 81, 146
vitamin, 38, 40, 149, 188–9, 190, 194
A, 40, 188
B, 40
C, 188
carotenoids, 188, 191–2, 194
E, 149
folate, 40, 105, 188
retinoids, 40, 188, 191–2, 194
vomiting, 117, 118, 198, 199
acute, 118, 119
anticipatory, 118
delayed, 118–19

war
First World War, 105
Second World War, 105, 140–1
Western blot, 57
wood dust, 37

x-rays, 43, 44, 51, 60, 61, 62–3, 65,
66, 68, 71, 72, 73, 77, 85, 95,
96, 98, 102, 152, 159
chest, 62–3, 171, 182
tomograph, 62, 71
xeroderma pigmentosum, 45, 191

yew, 107, 110